Health Services Research and Evidence-Based Medicine in Hand Surgery

Editors

JENNIFER F. WALJEE
KATE NELLANS

HAND CLINICS

www.hand.theclinics.com

Consulting Editor
KEVIN C. CHUNG

August 2014 • Volume 30 • Number 3

ELSEVIER

1600 John F. Kennedy Boulevard • Suite 1800 • Philadelphia, Pennsylvania, 19103-2899

http://www.theclinics.com

HAND CLINICS Volume 30, Number 3
August 2014 ISSN 0749-0712, ISBN-13: 978-0-323-32013-9

Editor: Jennifer Flynn-Briggs
Developmental editor: Stephanie Carter

Hand Clinics (ISSN 0749-0712) is published quarterly by Elsevier Inc., 360 Park Avenue South, New York, NY 10010-1710. Months of publication are February, May, August, and November. Business and Editorial Offices: 1600 John F. Kennedy Blvd., Ste. 1800, Philadelphia, PA 19103-2899. Customer Service Office: 3251 Riverport Lane, Maryland Heights, MO 63043. Periodicals postage paid at New York, NY and at additional mailing offices. Subscription price is $390.00 per year (domestic individuals), $606.00 per year (domestic institutions), $194.00 per year (domestic students/residents), $445.00 per year (Canadian individuals), $691.00 per year (Canadian institutions), $530.00 per year (international individuals), $691.00 per year (international institutions), and $256.00 per year (international and Canadian students/residents). Foreign air speed delivery is included in all *Clinics* subscription prices. All prices are subject to change without notice. **POSTMASTER:** Send address changes to *Hand Clinics*, Elsevier Health Sciences Division, Subscription Customer Service, 3251 Riverport Lane, Maryland Heights, MO 63043. Customer Service (orders, claims, online, change of address): Elsevier Health Sciences Division, Subscription Customer Service, 3251 Riverport Lane, Maryland Heights, MO 63043. Tel: 1-800-654-2452 (U.S. and Canada); 314-447-8871 (outside U.S. and Canada). Fax: 314-447-8029. E-mail: journalscustomerservice-usa@elsevier.com (for print support); journalsonlinesupport-usa@elsevier.com (for online support).

Reprints. For copies of 100 or more of articles in this publication, please contact the Commercial Reprints Department, Elsevier Inc., 360 Park Avenue South, New York, New York 10010-1710. Tel.: 212-633-3874; Fax: 212-633-3820; E-mail: reprints@elsevier.com.

Hand Clinics is covered in *MEDLINE/PubMed (Index Medicus), Current Contents/Clinical Medicine, EMBASE/Excerpta Medica,* and *ISI/BIOMED.*

Contributors

CONSULTING EDITOR

KEVIN C. CHUNG, MD, MS
Charles B.G.de Nancrede Professor
of Surgery, Section of Plastic Surgery,
Department of Surgery; Professor of
Orthopaedic Surgery; Assistant Dean for
Faculty Affairs; Associate Director of Global
REACH, University of Michigan Medical
School, University of Michigan Health
System, University of Michigan, Ann Arbor,
Michigan

EDITORS

JENNIFER F. WALJEE, MD, MS, MPH
Assistant Professor of Surgery, Section
of Plastic Surgery, Department of Surgery,
University of Michigan Medical School,
University of Michigan Medical Center,
University of Michigan Health System,
Ann Arbor, Michigan

KATE NELLANS, MD, MPH
Assistant Professor of Orthopedic Surgery,
Hofstra North Shore Long Island Jewish School
of Medicine, Great Neck, New York

AUTHORS

JOSHUA M. ADKINSON, MD
Fellow, Section of Plastic Surgery,
Department of Surgery, University of
Michigan Health System, Ann Arbor, Michigan

MOHIT BHANDARI, MD, PhD, FRCSC
Professor, Department of Clinical
Epidemiology and Biostatistics; Division of
Orthopaedic Surgery, Department of Surgery,
McMaster University, Hamilton, Ontario,
Canada

NANCY J.O. BIRKMEYER, PhD
Director, Michigan Bariatric Surgery
Collaborative; Senior Scientist, Center for
Healthcare Outcomes and Policy; Associate
Professor of Surgery, Department of Surgery,
University of Michigan Medical Center,
Ann Arbor, Michigan

JAMES CHANG, MD, FACS
Professor of Surgery (Plastic Surgery) &
Orthopedic Surgery; Chief, Division
of Plastic and Reconstructive Surgery,
Stanford University Medical Center,
Palo Alto, California

KEVIN C. CHUNG, MD, MS
Charles B.G.de Nancrede Professor
of Surgery, Section of Plastic Surgery,
Department of Surgery; Professor of
Orthopaedic Surgery; Assistant Dean for
Faculty Affairs; Associate Director of
Global REACH, University of Michigan
Medical School, University of Michigan
Health System, University of Michigan,
Ann Arbor, Michigan

CHRISTOPHER J. CORONEOS, MD
Resident, Division of Plastic and
Reconstructive Surgery, Department of
Surgery; Surgical Outcomes Research Centre
(SOURCE), McMaster University, Hamilton,
Ontario, Canada

CATHERINE CURTIN, MD
Assistant Professor of Plastic Surgery, Palo
Alto Veterans Hospital and Stanford University,
Palo Alto, California

REID W. DRAEGER, MD
Fellow, Mary S. Stern Hand Surgery
Fellowship, Department of Orthopaedic
Surgery, University of Cincinnati, Cincinnati,
Ohio

BRENT GRAHAM, MD, MSc, FRCSC
Assistant Professor, Hand Program,
Department of Surgery, University of Toronto,
University Health Network, Toronto, Ontario,
Canada

KENNETH HUI, BA
Section of Plastic Surgery, Division of Plastic
and Reconstructive Surgery, Stanford
University Medical Center, VA Palo Alto Health
Care System, Palo Alto, California

SHEPARD P. JOHNSON, MBBS
Resident, Department of Surgery, Saint Joseph
Mercy Hospital, Ann Arbor, Michigan

JOY C. MACDERMID, BScPT, PhD
School of Rehabilitation Sciences, McMaster
University, Hamilton; Clinical Research
Laboratory, Hand and Upper Limb Centre,
St. Joseph's Health Centre, London, Ontario,
Canada

**RORY B. MCGOLDRICK, MD, BSc (Hons),
FRCS(Plast), MBA**
Postdoctoral Research Scholar, Section
of Plastic Surgery, Division of Plastic and
Reconstructive Surgery, Stanford University
Medical Center, VA Palo Alto Health Care
System, Palo Alto, California

KATE NELLANS, MD, MPH
Assistant Professor of Orthopedic Surgery,
Hofstra North Shore Long Island Jewish School
of Medicine, Great Neck, New York

ERIKA D. SEARS, MD, MS
Hand Surgery Fellow, Section of Plastic
Surgery, Department of Surgery, The
University of Michigan Health System, Ann
Arbor, Michigan

LEE SQUITIERI, MD, MS
Resident Physician, Division of Plastic and
Reconstructive Surgery, Department of
Surgery, University of Southern California,
Los Angeles, California

PETER J. STERN, MD
Professor; Director, Mary S. Stern Hand
Surgery Fellowship, Department of
Orthopaedic Surgery, University of
Cincinnati, Cincinnati, Ohio

ROBERT M. SZABO, MD, MPH
Professor of Orthopaedic and Plastic Surgery;
Chief of Hand and Microvascular Surgery;
Director of Hand and Upper Extremity Surgery
Fellowship, Department of Orthopaedic
Surgery, University of California, Davis,
Sacramento, California

**ACHILLEAS THOMA, MD, MSc, FRCSC,
FACS**
Professor, Division of Plastic and
Reconstructive Surgery, Department of
Surgery; Surgical Outcomes Research Centre
(SOURCE); Department of Clinical
Epidemiology and Biostatistics, McMaster
University, Hamilton, Ontario, Canada

SOPHOCLES H. VOINESKOS, MD, MSc
Resident, Division of Plastic and
Reconstructive Surgery, Department of
Surgery; Surgical Outcomes Research Centre
(SOURCE), McMaster University, Hamilton,
Ontario, Canada

JENNIFER F. WALJEE, MD, MS, MPH
Assistant Professor of Surgery, Section of
Plastic Surgery, Department of Surgery,
University of Michigan Medical School,
University of Michigan Medical Center,
University of Michigan Health System,
Ann Arbor, Michigan

BRIAN ZAFONTE, MD, PhD
Orthopaedic Hand and Upper Extremity
Surgery Fellow, Department of Orthopaedic
Surgery, University of California, Davis,
Sacramento, California

Contents

Preface: Evidence-based Medicine in Hand Surgery   xi

Jennifer F. Waljee and Kate Nellans

Health Services Research: Evolution and Applications   259

Kate Nellans and Jennifer F. Waljee

> Health services research (HSR) is broadly focused on characterizing and improving the access, quality, delivery, and cost of health care. HSR is a multidisciplinary field, engaging experts in clinical medicine and surgery, policy, economics, implementation science, statistics, psychology, and education to improve the care of patients across all specialties. This article summarizes the evolution and distinctive attributes of HSR and present several real-world applications.

Evidence-Based Medicine in Hand Surgery: Clinical Applications and Future Direction   269

Brian Zafonte and Robert M. Szabo

> Evidence-based medicine empowers physicians to systematically analyze published data so as to quickly formulate treatment plans that deliver safe, robust, and cost-effective patient care. In this article, we sample some areas in hand and upper extremity surgery where the evidence base is strong enough that it has or should have unified treatment strategies; we identify some problems where good evidence has failed to unify treatment, and discuss problems for which evidence is still lacking but needed because treatment remains controversial. We also discuss circumstances in which level 4 evidence is more likely than randomized trials to guide treatment.

Measuring and Understanding Treatment Effectiveness in Hand Surgery   285

Sophocles H. Voineskos, Christopher J. Coroneos, Achilleas Thoma, and Mohit Bhandari

> Incorporating evidence-based medicine into practice is now an expectation for hand surgeons. Hand surgeons need to be able to assess associated benefits, risks, cost, and applicability of a treatment option when providing care to their patients. Using a clinical example, this article takes the reader through the three-step approach when using a publication from the medical literature on therapy. The focus of this article is primarily the second and third steps, which involve measuring and understanding treatment effectiveness.

Patient-Reported Outcomes: State-of-the-Art Hand Surgery and Future Applications   293

Joy C. MacDermid

> Patient-reported outcome measures (PRO) can provide reliable and valid estimates of patient status and response to interventions to complete the final step in an evidence-based patient interaction. A variety of PRO are relevant to upper extremity surgery and rehabilitation outcomes. PRO provide feasible tools for clinical research or practice, although use in clinical decision making lags behind research applications. Recent trends in clinical measurement include better integration of International Classification of Functioning, Disability and Health in content validation, more modern methods of evaluating scaling properties (Rasch analysis), consensus exercise on establishing core measures, electronic data collection, and computer-adaptive testing.

Bench to Bedside: Integrating Advances in Basic Science into Daily Clinical Practice   305

Rory B. McGoldrick, Kenneth Hui, and James Chang

This article focuses on the initial steps of commercial development of a patentable scientific discovery from an academic center through to marketing a clinical product. The basics of partnering with a technology transfer office (TTO) and the complex process of patenting are addressed, followed by a discussion on marketing and licensing the patent to a company in addition to starting a company. Finally, the authors address the basic principles of obtaining clearance from the Food and Drugs Administration, production in a good manufacturing practice (GMP) facility, and bringing the product to clinical trial.

Comparative Effectiveness Research in Hand Surgery   319

Shepard P. Johnson and Kevin C. Chung

Comparative effectiveness research (CER) is a concept initiated by the Institute of Medicine and financially supported by the federal government. The primary objective of CER is to improve decision making in medicine. This research is intended to evaluate the effectiveness, benefits, and harmful effects of alternative interventions. CER studies are commonly large, simple, observational, and conducted using electronic databases. To date, there is little comparative effectiveness evidence within hand surgery to guide therapeutic decisions. To draw conclusions on effectiveness through electronic health records, databases must contain clinical information and outcomes relevant to hand surgery interventions, such as patient-related outcomes.

Quality Assessment in Hand Surgery   329

Jennifer F. Waljee and Catherine Curtin

Measuring quality assessment in hand surgery remains an underexplored area. However, measuring quality is becoming increasingly transparent and important. Patients now have direct access to hospital and physician metrics and large payers have linked financial incentives to quality metrics. It is critical for hand surgeons to understand the essential elements of quality and its assessment. This article reviews several areas of hand surgery quality assessments including safety, outcomes, satisfaction, and cost.

Collaborative Quality Improvement in Surgery   335

Jennifer F. Waljee and Nancy J.O. Birkmeyer

Collaborative quality improvement has demonstrated success in improving quality and reducing health care costs in several state-based examples. Professional societies and payers are keen on identifying the most effective strategies to improve the safety and efficiency of surgical care. This review highlights the development and features of collaborative quality improvement programs, their advantages and examples of successful collaborations for several surgical conditions, and their potential application for surgeons caring for patients with upper extremity trauma and disability.

The Patient Protection and Affordable Care Act: A Primer for Hand Surgeons   345

Joshua M. Adkinson and Kevin C. Chung

The Affordable Care Act is the largest and most comprehensive overhaul of the United States health care industry since the inception of the Medicare and Medicaid.

Contained within the 10 titles are a multitude of provisions that will change how hand surgeons practice medicine and how they are reimbursed. It is imperative that surgeons are equipped with the knowledge of how this law will affect all physician practices and hospitals.

Patient-Centered Care in Medicine and Surgery: Guidelines for Achieving Patient-Centered Subspecialty Care
353

Reid W. Draeger and Peter J. Stern

Patient-centered care is based on the principle that equality between physician and patient is mutually advantageous. This model of care recently has largely supplanted the historical paternalistic model of the physician-patient relationship. Patient-centered care differs from the disease-centered model of evidence-based medicine, but the two are not mutually exclusive. Patient-centered care has 5 core components: the biopsychosocial perspective, the patient as person, sharing power and responsibility, the therapeutic alliance, and the doctor as person. This article explores these components, explains the differences between patient-centered care and evidence-based medicine, and offers guidelines for achieving patient-centered subspecialty care in hand surgery.

Clinical Practice Guidelines: What Are They and How Should They Be Disseminated?   361

Brent Graham

Clinical practice guidelines summarize the available evidence for patient management in a format that is easy for clinicians to use. These guidelines usually use methodologically rigorous principles for retrieving and evaluating the literature and for establishing consensus among work group members, but implementation by clinicians is often incomplete. The reasons why guidelines fail to gain widespread acceptance vary with the topic and clinician group. Successful dissemination of practice guidelines requires an understanding of the barriers to implementation and the use of multiple strategies to address these. This article examines the factors affecting implementation and the approaches to overcoming these obstacles.

Funding Research in the Twenty-First Century: Current Opinions and Future Directions
367

Lee Squitieri and Kevin C. Chung

For all academic biomedical researchers, the process of submitting grants and securing research funding is a critical part of advancing one's career. In the current era of decreasing new grant awards and renewals leading to significantly worse success rates, it is hard for young aspiring physician-scientists to remain optimistic regarding their future in academic medicine. It is important that today's young surgeon-scientists prepare for and adapt to the inevitably changing climate of research funding. This article provides a primer on developing a successful career as a funded surgeon-scientist and pathways for building a robust research platform worthy of extramural National Institutes of Health funding in the twenty-first century.

Future Education and Practice Initiatives in Hand Surgery: Improving Fulfillment of Patient Needs
377

Erika D. Sears and Kevin C. Chung

In the current health care environment, there are several areas in the delivery of health care to patients having hand surgery that need improvement to adequately fulfill patient needs, including difficulty in maintaining adequate emergency call coverage for patients having hand surgery, decreasing trends in hand surgeons willing to perform microsurgery and replantation, and deficiencies in musculoskeletal education of non–hand surgery providers. Both educational reforms and reforms in the practice environment are needed to improve the ability of hand surgeons to fulfill patient needs in the future.

Index   **387**

HAND CLINICS

FORTHCOMING ISSUES

November 2014
Options for Surgical Exposure and Soft Tissue Coverage in Upper Extremity Trauma
Amitava Gupta, *Editor*

February 2015
New Developments in Management of Vascular Pathology of the Upper Extremity
Steven Moran, Karim Bakri, and James Higgins, *Editors*

RECENT ISSUES

May 2014
Flap Reconstruction of the Traumatized Upper Extremity
Kevin C. Chung, *Editor*

February 2014
Minimally Invasive Hand Surgery
Catherine Curtin, *Editor*

November 2013
Management of Hand Fractures
Jeffrey N. Lawton, *Editor*

August 2013
Peripheral Nerve Conditions: Using Evidence to Guide Treatment
Warren C. Hammert, *Editor*

Preface
Evidence-based Medicine in Hand Surgery

We are honored to serve as guest editors of this issue of *Hand Clinics*, which is focused on the integration of health services research into clinical practice. Our goal is to provide an overview of the field of health services research for the practicing hand surgeon and to highlight pertinent topics that can inform clinical care in any practice setting. We have chosen health services research topics from three broad areas: scientific investigation, quality of care, and health care policy. The authors featured in this issue have provided a closer look at several key topics, such as evidence-based practice, patient-centered care, translating research in into practice, and health care reform. We are pleased to have gathered the perspectives of pioneers and leaders in this field of research to understand how these concepts can be applied to the practice of Hand Surgery.

We greatly appreciate the contributions of each author. We would also like to thank Stephanie Carter and Jennifer Flynn-Briggs at Elsevier for their hard work and enthusiasm during the creation of this edition. Finally, we are incredibly grateful to our mentor, Dr Kevin Chung, who has given us the opportunity to lead this issue of *Hand Clinics*. He has steadfastly guided us during our training, and now as young hand surgeons in practice. His unwavering dedication to improving the practice of Hand Surgery through health services research is unmatched and inspires us to critically assess our practices daily and to continually strive for excellence as we care for our patients.

Thank you,
Jennifer and Kate

Jennifer F. Waljee, MD, MS, MPH
Section of Plastic Surgery
Department of Surgery
University of Michigan Medical Center
1500 East Medical Center Drive
Ann Arbor, MI 48103, USA

Kate Nellans, MD, MPH
Orthopedic Surgery
Hofstra North Shore Long Island Jewish
School of Medicine
611 Northern Boulevard, Suite 200
Great Neck, NY 11021, USA

E-mail addresses:
filip@med.umich.edu (J.F. Waljee)
katy.nellans@gmail.com (K. Nellans)

Health Services Research
Evolution and Applications

Kate Nellans, MD, MPH[a], Jennifer F. Waljee, MD, MS, MPH[b],*

KEYWORDS

- Health services research • Outcomes research • Health care quality

KEY POINTS

- Health services research is broadly focused on characterizing and improving the access, quality, delivery, and cost of health care.
- Health services research is a multidisciplinary field, engaging experts in clinical medicine and surgery, policy, economics, implementation science, statistics, psychology, and education to improve the care of patients across all specialties.
- Recent health policy changes emphasize the need for rigorous, ongoing assessment of our health care delivery system. Health services research endeavors will become increasingly relevant with accelerating health care costs, medical and surgical innovation, and the expanding population in the United States.

INTRODUCTION

Delivering high-quality, efficient care to all Americans remains an elusive and expensive task. Understanding the organizational structure of our health care delivery system can provide critical insight on strategies to improve the accessibility, effectiveness, and affordability of health care in the United States. In this context, the field of health services research (HSR) is directed at examining all aspects of health care delivery to improve the quality and streamline the allocation of scare resources. This article summarizes the evolution and distinctive attributes of HSR and present several real-world applications.

THE HISTORY OF HEALTH SERVICES RESEARCH

The beginning of HSR as a formal entity is difficult to define. For example, the first investigation of treatment effectiveness could be considered as early as biblical times. In the Book of Daniel, King Nebuchadnezzar of Babylon decreed that only wine and meat should be consumed to maintain health and prevent disease.[1] Early examples of evidence-based medicine can also be found in the first century AD, when members of the Song dynasty advocated the health benefits of ginseng through comparative, albeit anecdotal, accounts.[2] Regardless of its true beginning, throughout history, there are innumerable examples of efforts to identify best practices and improve the delivery of health care. For example, in 1789, the Public Health Service was established as a strategy to ensure appropriate care was given to ailing or injured merchant seamen in the United States.[3] In 1837, William Farr collected statistical data regarding mortality, morbidity, and disability. Florence Nightingale furthered this work in 1858 with Farr, developing a uniform reporting system of health care practices and outcomes for London Hospitals.[4]

In the United States, HSR formalized during the mid-twentieth century following medical and

The authors have nothing to disclose.
[a] Hofstra North Shore Long Island Jewish School of Medicine, 611 Northern Boulevard, Suite 200, Great Neck, NY 11021, USA; [b] Section of Plastic Surgery, University of Michigan Medical School, 1500 East Medical Center Drive, Ann Arbor, MI 48109-5340, USA
* Corresponding author. Section of Plastic Surgery, University of Michigan Health System, 2130 Taubman Center, SPC 5340, 1500 East Medical Center Drive, Ann Arbor, MI 48109-5340.
E-mail address: filip@umich.edu

Hand Clin 30 (2014) 259–268
http://dx.doi.org/10.1016/j.hcl.2014.05.004
0749-0712/14/$ – see front matter © 2014 Elsevier Inc. All rights reserved.

technological advances from World War I and World War II.[5] Before this, medical care was relatively accessible and inexpensive in the United States. However, effective treatments were lacking for many conditions, such as common infections or pregnancy complications. Military conflict spurred the development of numerous advances in medical and surgical diagnosis and treatment, such as blood transfusions, antisepsis, radiographs, electrocardiograms, and triage systems.[4] This explosion of innovation was correlated with not only a rapid decline in morbidity and mortality but also a sharp increase in expenditures, prompting a closer examination of health care delivery.

The term "health services research" was formally coined in 1966.[3] At that time, the federal government established a specific study section for grant proposals that were health services oriented.[3] In 1968, the National Center for Health Services Research and Development was established under the leadership of Dr Kerr White, a pioneer in HSR in the mid-twentieth century. The National Center for Health Services Research, known today as the Agency for Healthcare Research and Quality (AHRQ), represents one of the first federally funded programs charged with systematically examining health care delivery and quality in the United States. HSR gained further momentum with the appropriation of research funds specific to the purpose of advancing the field of HSR, spearheaded by Dr Paul Sanazaro.[5] Today, AHRQ is the primary federal agency focused on the delivery of health care in the United States and funds most of the HSR in the United States. With an annual operating budget of approximately 400 million dollars, more than 80% is directed toward HSR-related grants and contacts and more than 12,000 active health services researchers in the United States.[6]

WHAT IS HEALTH SERVICES RESEARCH?

HSR has been broadly defined as the study of health care access, cost, and effectiveness, with the purpose of developing successful strategies to organize, manage, finance, and deliver high-quality medical care.[5,7] HSR has expanded dramatically to become a multidisciplinary field in which investigators study health care delivery. Collaborators include specialists from clinical medicine, economics, psychology, statistics, education, and policy. With rapid advances in measurement technique, study design, and information technology, HSR has profoundly shaped health care delivery in the United States in the twentieth and twenty-first centuries.

ASPECTS OF HEALTH SERVICES RESEARCH

In general, HSR involves the examination of the effect of specific aspects of the health care system on endpoints, such as clinical outcomes (eg, mortality), quality of life (eg, pain), or cost. **Fig. 1** describes a thematic overview of HSR. Nearly all HSR endeavors examine topics in 1 of 3 broad categories—access to care, quality of care, or cost of care—and seek to affect change in the following avenues: outcomes, policy, or system delivery. HSR uses a variety of study methods to accomplish these goals, which are outlined in **Table 1**. Although not an absolutely inclusive or comprehensive list, HSR studies generally include methodology, access to care, efficacy, quality, cost, or evaluation of effectiveness.

Methodology studies identify the strategies for measuring aspects or characteristics of the health care system. For example, in 2004, the National Institutes of Health has initiated collaborative efforts to improve HRQOL measurement using common data elements and develop a universal metric for comparison across conditions, called Patient-Reported Outcomes Measurement Information System (PROMIS).[8,9] Such tools can allow researchers and policy makers capture the outcomes most relevant to patients in an accurate and reliable way. Other examples include identifying tools to capture important outcomes, such

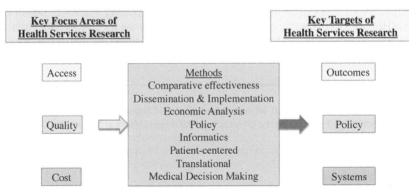

Fig. 1. Thematic overview of health services research.

Table 1
Examples of health services research

Type	Definition	Examples
Method	Research that focuses on strategies or methods to examine aspects of the health care system	Creating instruments to measure quality of life[9] Creating risk and reliability models to compare outcomes across providers[55]
Access	Research that examines the ability of individuals to engage the health care system appropriately	Racial disparities in specialist referral and treatment outcomes[89,90] Socioeconomic disparities in access to dental care[91]
Efficacy	Research that examines the ability of a diagnostic tool treatment or other intervention to change an outcome	Randomized controlled trial examining efficacy of distal radius fracture treatment[92] Randomized controlled trial of vitamin C on the prevention of regional pain syndrome following fracture[93]
Quality	Research that examines the effectiveness and safety of the care delivered to individuals	Does selective referral of patients to centers of excellence reduce complication rates?[94] Do hospitals differ in their ability to "rescue" patients from complications?[43]
Cost	Research that examines health care expenditures or costs with or without comparison of benefits	Cost-utility analysis of treatment of Dupuytren contractures in the hand[95] Projected costs of distal radius fractures among the elderly[96]
Evaluation	Research that examines clinical practice in a "real-world" setting or the effectiveness of health system interventions on care	The effect of national policy on rates of surgery, such as breast reconstruction[97] The effect of Medicaid expansion on subspecialty procedures[98] Ethnographic techniques to define the "root cause" of surgical complications[10,35]

as post-operative complications, or analyze outcomes and place findings into an appropriate context.[10–12]

Most commonly, HSR focuses on studies of treatment effectiveness. Efficacy describes the extent to which a treatment yields its intended effect under ideal circumstances, and efficacy trials are those in which the effects of a specific treatment option are examined in a well-controlled setting with a homogeneous population to examine its performance under ideal conditions.[13] These trials are often performed early on in the development of a medical treatment, such as in animal models or small cohorts of highly selected individuals. In an efficacy trial, validity should be maximized because potential sources of bias or confounding can modify the estimates between cause and effect is minimized. Randomized controlled trials are considered the gold standard for describing the effectiveness of a treatment and provide the highest level of evidence of causality.[14–16] Despite their advantages, randomized controlled trials are expensive and labor intensive. It is essential to include a sample of adequate size to achieve sufficient power without expending additional funds for unnecessary observations. Clinical trials also require extensive collaboration, organization, and commitment often across multiple centers. Finally, generalizability may be limited in controlled trials due to the stringency of exclusion and inclusion criteria.[17]

In contrast to efficacy, effectiveness is the ability for a treatment to achieve its intended effect in a typical clinical setting. For example, a drug may be very effective in a cadaver model, or in a selected group of individuals, but does not translate into clinical success. Treatments may not be implemented due to barriers such as provider bias and uncertainty, poor access to health care resources, and patient factors and preferences.[18] Unlike efficacy trials, effectiveness studies measure treatment outcomes in the context of patient factors, societal factors, and health care structure and process.[19,20] Although there may be more inherent "noise" in such trials because of greater heterogeneity, effectiveness studies provide more robust measures of treatment effects, providing insight on barriers and facilitators to treatment implementation.

In addition to treatment effectiveness, HSR studies may focus more directly on health care utilization and access to care and identify important disparities. Utilization of health care can include primary care provider visits, emergency care, subspecialist referral, or post-acute care rehabilitation needs. For example, an analysis of administrative data revealed significant disparities in amputation rates by race among patients with peripheral vascular occlusive disease. Furthermore, differences in disease severity at the time of presentation for many conditions may represent profoundly different access to specialist care and disease screening resources.[21,22] Administrative data can also be leveraged to examine health care expenditures. For example, Medicare spending varies widely across the United States, even after price adjustment analysis.[23] These differences are not borne evenly by providers, and differences highlight opportunities to streamline care and achieve better value in care.[24,25]

Defining quality is a fundamental aspect of HSR. One of the oldest, and most widely used, frameworks of HSR was described by Donabedian, which relates the factors that contribute to quality of care (**Fig. 2**). In this framework, structure includes those variables that describe the setting of health care delivery, such as the facility, available resources, and human resources (surgeon training and expertise).[26–28] Process of care variables describe aspects of care and clinical practice that patients receive, such as perioperative beta blockage or the use of sequential compression devices or unfractionated heparin to reduce the risk of perioperative venous thromboembolism. Finally, in this model, outcomes describe the end results from treatment. These end results can include clinical events, such as mortality or complication rates, cost, patient-reported outcomes, or patient experiences (eg, satisfaction). In HSR, each of these components has been leveraged to create strategies for quality assessment improvement.[4] For example, hospitals with greater care capacity, technologic advances, and teaching facilities were correlated with greater ability to rescue patients from major post-operative complications.[29] Understanding these correlates of improved outcomes can inform strategies to improve overall surgical care.

Although large, population-based studies can provide robust data regarding the quality of care, and studies that evaluate the nuances of cause and effect can provide rich information regarding the delivery of care. For example, qualitative methods facilitate in-depth exploration of topics about which little is known and may therefore better elucidate functional and aesthetic outcomes by revealing patients' perspectives in their own words without the restrictions of survey answer choices.[18,19] Qualitative studies can capture phenomena, such as attitudes, value systems, cultural mores, and motivations that are difficult to measure quantitatively because it is constrained by investigator-selected criteria.[30–32] For example, Aravind and colleagues[33] conducted semistructured interviews with 20 patients who suffered from open type IIIB or IIIC lower extremity traumatic injuries to examine and determine the effect of amputation or reconstruction on health-related quality of life.[30] Using qualitative methods, the investigators effectively present a cognitive framework for the psychosocial components of recovery and post-operative disability. Such data can highlight unmet patient needs and be applied toward developing quantitative instruments to measure patient-reported outcomes. Ethnographic studies can provide a root-cause analysis of the factors that result in post-operative complications.[34] For example, Symons and colleagues[35] followed patients who had undergone surgery to identify failures in processes of care. In this study, trained observers recorded post-operative events among 50 patients who underwent routine surgical procedures. In this study, most failures were preventable, more than half resulting in patient harm, and were primarily due to communication breakdowns or delays in care.

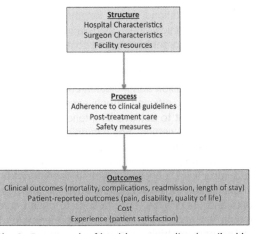

Fig. 2. Framework of health care quality described by Donabedian. (*Data from* Donabedian A. Evaluating the quality of medical care. Milbank Mem Fund Q 1966;44:166–206.)

HEALTH SERVICES RESEARCH IN SURGERY: PRACTICAL EXAMPLES

In 2001, the Institute of Medicine defined the standards by which health care delivery in the United States should be considered. In *Crossing the Quality Chiasm: A New Healthcare System for the 21st Century,* the IOM laid out 6 critical elements: (1) safety, (2) effectiveness, (3) cost-efficient, (4) accessible, (5) patient-centered, and (6) equity.[36] In the field of surgery, the HSR movement has examined the delivery of care by each of these standards and made important contributions in defining variation in care, outcomes assessment, and patient engagement in procedural care.

Variation in Care

Led by John Wennberg, the Dartmouth Institute for Health Policy and Clinical Practice has systematically evaluated variation in medical and surgical care in the United States across a wide range of disciplines over the last 30 years.[37] The Dartmouth Atlas of Health care (www.dartmouthatlas.org) describes regional differences in the delivery of care, utilization of care, and spending for common conditions and procedures, such as tonsillectomy, joint replacement, major cardiovascular procedures, and general surgery procedures (eg, mastectomy, cholecystectomy). Although variation in care could be attributable to chance alone, wide disparities in care more likely signal important differences in health care quality, including the overuse, underuse, and misuse of resources.[26,38] A closer look reveals that most differences in health care spending can be attributed to differences in health care utilization. However, care is not accessed proportionally by need (ie, sicker patients do not always receive more health care), and differences in health care spending do not correlate with improved outcomes in the United States.[37,39]

Building on this work in surgery, health services researchers have been instrumental in defining those factors that explain variation in surgical performance or why some hospitals and surgeons achieve better outcomes than others. For example, Birkmeyer and colleagues[40–42] have demonstrated a clear, causal relationship between experience and outcomes. Their work using population-based administrative data reveals that hospitals and surgeons who more commonly perform procedures achieve better outcomes for many common procedures. Furthermore, providers who have more experience with procedures are better equipped to deal with surgical complications.[43] Finally, differences in performance and skill at the surgeon level are measurable and correlated with differences in procedural outcomes.[44] This

seminal work has provided a framework for examining provider performance on a population-based level across many disciplines.[45–50]

Capturing Post-operative Outcomes: How and What to Measure

Quality measures typically compare post-operative clinical outcomes, such as 30-day mortality, readmission, or complication rates (eg, venous thromboembolism). However, to accurately assess performance using outcomes, it is essential to control for differences in case mix across providers.[26] For example, large, tertiary care referral hospitals more frequently perform complex procedures due to differences in hospital infrastructure and available resources. Furthermore, patient clinical and sociodemographic characteristics vary widely among providers. In surgery, multiple approaches have been proposed for risk adjustment and can be applied at the patient level.[51–54] However, the specific variables and number of variables remain an area of ongoing exploration.[53] In addition to risk adjustment, clinical outcomes can be further refined using reliability adjustment. Random variation due to small sample sizes can introduce statistical "noise" into estimates and limit the power to detect variation across hospitals. Reliability adjustment can substantially influence performance assessment and yield more accurate comparisons.[55]

Quality assessment can be further improved by the use of composite measures of performance to provide a more comprehensive perspective of performance. Composite measures combine multiple indicators of quality that are relevant to a condition or procedure of interest. For example, Dimick and colleagues[56] have created a composite measure of quality combining mortality, reoperation, length of stay, and morbidity indicators to assess outcomes following common surgical procedures. Compared with single risk-adjusted measures of performance, such as mortality, composite measures are better predictors of outcomes following surgery. Composite measures have been successfully applied for key conditions, including myocardial infarction and pneumonia, and are increasingly applied toward surgical care.[57–59]

However, even when optimally risk and reliability-adjusted outcomes are available, these endpoints may be insensitive for certain procedures. For example, most many procedures in hand surgery are performed to improve symptoms and function, with relatively few readmissions and minimal mortality or serious morbidity risk. Therefore, it is difficult to measure performance precisely based on rare events.[60,61] Patient-reported outcomes, such as pain, disability, and social functioning, could provide a more accurate assessment of treatment effectiveness and performance, but are rarely collected in a systematic way, and not typically available on a population-based level in the United States. In the United Kingdom and Sweden, patient-reported outcomes are routinely collected following common surgical procedures and will provide a framework for the implementation of patient-centered quality assessment and improvement going forward in the United States.[62–70]

Patient Engagement in Surgery

In addition to differences in performance, variation in rates of surgery may represent differences in the involvement of the patient in the decision for surgery.[71,72] For example, geographic variation in mastectomy rates has prompted concerns that women are not uniformly counseled regarding the surgical treatment of early-stage breast cancer.[73–76] In the early twentieth century, the patient-doctor relationship was largely viewed as paternalistic one, with most of the responsibility for clinical decision making resting on physicians. More recently, patients have been redefined as consumers and are empowered to participate in the decision for care, particularly in those situations in which treatment outcomes may be equivocal.[77] Although the Internet has dramatically expanded the information that patients have available to them when making health care choices, the accuracy of available resources and their effect on patient knowledge remains inconsistent.[78–81] Recently, efforts have been directed on developing and incorporating decision aids and support tools into routine care to help describe surgical risk, details of surgical procedures, and indications for intervention. In this way, HSR has identified pathways to engage patients in their surgical care and improve the decision-making process.[71,82,83]

HEALTH SERVICES RESEARCH IN HAND SURGERY

Recent events in health care reform in the United States underscore the need for robust HSR efforts to critically evaluate and improve our health care system. However, the field of hand surgery is a particularly challenging substrate for HSR. The procedures that encompass hand surgery are diverse and nuanced, such as the surgical management of thumb carpometacarpal arthritis or the fixation of distal radius fractures. Furthermore, relative to other conditions, such as obesity, heart disease, and diabetes, many hand maladies are uncommon, such as ulnar impaction, Dupuytren

disease, and congenital hand differences. Although the authors' subspecialty journals have adopted level of evidence standards, a paucity of high level of evidence studies persists, and there is variable implementation of available data in clinical practice.[14,84–88] Finally, hand surgery is relatively safe, with few associated readmissions and low rates of mortality. Therefore, measures of disability, pain, and function are ideal outcomes, but often difficult to capture on a broad level. Nonetheless, the lessons and examples in HSR in other fields, such as general surgery, cardiology, and primary care, can serve as a template for improving the delivery of hand surgery going forward.

In this issue of Hand Clinics, the authors examine several aspects of HSR in more detail to provide a framework and foundation for future efforts to this end in the area of upper extremity care. First, they examine strategies to optimize scientific investigation, including the integration of patient-reported outcomes into research, standards for measuring treatment effectiveness, translating research findings into clinical practice, the principles of comparative effectiveness research, and conceptualizing the evidence available for the practice of upper extremity surgery. They then consider how health care quality can be measured in hand surgery and examine the integration of collaborative quality assessment and improvement in surgery on a population level. Finally, the authors highlight several important health care policy topics in hand surgery, including the development and implementation of clinical guidelines, patient-centered care in hand surgery, the financial infrastructure of health services research support, access to upper extremity care, and the current state and future directions of health care reform.

REFERENCES

1. Bhatt A. Evolution of clinical research: a history before and beyond James Lind. Perspect Clin Res 2010;1(1):6–10.
2. Claridge JA, Fabian TC. History and development of evidence-based medicine. World J Surg 2005; 29(5):547–53.
3. Bindman AB. The evolution of health services research. Health Serv Res 2013;48(2 Pt 1):349–53.
4. Steinwachs DM, Hughes RG. Health services research: scope and significance. In: Quality AFHRA, editor. Patient safety and quality: an evidence-based Handook for Nurses. 2008.
5. Lohr KN, Steinwachs DM. Health services research: an evolving definition of the field. Health Serv Res 2002;37(1):7–9.

6. McGinnis S, Moore J. The health services research workforce: current stock. Health Serv Res 2009; 44(6):2214–26.

7. Institute of Medicine, editor. Improving information services for health services researchers: a report to the library of medicine. Washington, DC: National Academy Press; 1991. Harris-Wehling J, Morris LS, editors. Board on Health Care Services.

8. Cella DF, Yount S, Rothrock N, et al. The Patient-Reported Outcomes Measurement Information System (PROMIS): progress of an NIH Roadmap cooperative group during its first two years. Med Care 2007;45(5 Suppl 1):S3–11.

9. Cella DF, Riley W, Stone A, et al. The Patient-Reported Outcomes Measurement Information System (PROMIS) developed and tested in its first wave of adult self-reported health outcome item banks: 2005-2008. J Clin Epidemiol 2010;63: 1179–94.

10. Waljee JF, Windisch S, Finks JF, et al. Classifying cause of death after cancer surgery. Surg Innov 2006;13(4):274–9.

11. Hayward RA, Heisler M, Adams J, et al. Overestimating outcome rates: statistical estimation when reliability is suboptimal. Health Serv Res 2007; 42(4):1718–38.

12. Smith KA, Sussman JB, Bernstein SJ, et al. Improving the reliability of physician "report cards". Med Care 2013;51(3):266–74.

13. Flay BR. Efficacy and effectiveness trials (and other phases of research) in the development of health promotion programs. Prev Med 1986;15(5):451–74.

14. Chung KC, Swanson JA, Schmitz D, et al. Introducing evidence-based medicine to plastic and reconstructive surgery. Plast Reconstr Surg 2009; 123(4):1385–9.

15. Burns PB, Rohrich RJ, Chung KC. The levels of evidence and their role in evidence-based medicine. Plast Reconstr Surg 2011;128(1):305–10.

16. Lipsky MS, Sharp LK. From idea to market: the drug approval process. J Am Board Fam Pract 2001;14(5):362–7.

17. Guyatt GH, Sinclair J, Cook DJ, et al. Users' guides to the medical literature: XVI. How to use a treatment recommendation. Evidence-Based Medicine Working Group and the Cochrane Applicability Methods Working Group. JAMA 1999;281(19): 1836–43.

18. El-Serag HB, Talwalkar J, Kim WR. Efficacy, effectiveness, and comparative effectiveness in liver disease. Hepatology 2010;52(2):403–7.

19. Steckler A, McLeroy KR. The importance of external validity. Am J Public Health 2008;98(1):9–10.

20. Gartlehner G, Hansen RA, Nissman D, et al. A simple and valid tool distinguished efficacy from effectiveness studies. J Clin Epidemiol 2006; 59(10):1040–8.

21. Morris AM, Billingsley KG, Baxter NN, et al. Racial disparities in rectal cancer treatment: a population-based analysis. Arch Surg 2004;139(2):151–5 [discussion: 156].

22. Hayanga AJ, Waljee AK, Kaiser HE, et al. Racial clustering and access to colorectal surgeons, gastroenterologists, and radiation oncologists by African Americans and Asian Americans in the United States: a county-level data analysis. Arch Surg 2009;144(6):532–5.

23. Gottlieb DJ, Zhou W, Song Y, et al. Prices don't drive regional Medicare spending variations. Health Aff 2010;29(3):537–43.

24. Miller DC, Gust C, Dimick JB, et al. Large variations in Medicare payments for surgery highlight savings potential from bundled payment programs. Health Aff (Millwood) 2011;30(11):2107–15.

25. Birkmeyer JD, Gust C, Baser O, et al. Medicare payments for common inpatient procedures: implications for episode-based payment bundling. Health Serv Res 2010;45(6 Pt 1):1783–95.

26. Birkmeyer JD, Dimick JB. Understanding and reducing variation in surgical mortality. Annu Rev Med 2009;60:405–15.

27. Birkmeyer JD, Dimick JB, Birkmeyer NJ. Measuring the quality of surgical care: structure, process, or outcomes? J Am Coll Surg 2004; 198(4):626–32.

28. Donabedian A. The quality of care. How can it be assessed? JAMA 1988;260(12):1743–8.

29. Ghaferi AA, Osborne NH, Birkmeyer JD, et al. Hospital characteristics associated with failure to rescue from complications after pancreatectomy. J Am Coll Surg 2010;211(3):325–30.

30. Shauver MS, Aravind MS, Chung KC. A Qualitative Study of Recovery From Type III-B and III-C Tibial Fractures. Ann Plast Surg 2011;66(1):73–9.

31. Shauver MJ, Chung KC. A guide to qualitative research in plastic surgery. Plast Reconstr Surg 2010;126(3):1089–97.

32. Hamill R, Carson S, Dorahy M. Experiences of psychosocial adjustment within 18 months of amputation: an interpretative phenomenological analysis. Disabil Rehabil 2010;32(9):729–40.

33. Aravind M, Shauver MJ, Chung KC. A qualitative analysis of the decision-making process for patients with severe lower leg trauma. Plast Reconstr Surg 2010;126(6):2019–29.

34. Greenberg CC, Regenbogen SE, Studdert DM, et al. Patterns of communication breakdowns resulting in injury to surgical patients. J Am Coll Surg 2007;204(4):533–40.

35. Symons NR, Almoudaris AM, Nagpal K, et al. An observational study of the frequency, severity, and etiology of failures in postoperative care after major elective general surgery. Ann Surg 2013; 257(1):1–5.

36. Institute of Medicine (U.S.). Committee on Quality of Health Care in America. Crossing the quality chasm: a new health system for the 21st century. Washington, DC: National Academy Press; 2001.

37. Fisher ES, Bynum JP, Skinner JS. Slowing the growth of health care costs–lessons from regional variation. N Engl J Med 2009;360(9):849–52.

38. Institute of Medicine. Crossing the quality chiasm: a new healthcare for the 21st centruy. 2001.

39. Weinstein MC, Skinner JA. Comparative effectiveness and health care spending–implications for reform. N Engl J Med 2010;362(5):460–5.

40. Birkmeyer JD, Dimick JB, Staiger DO. Operative mortality and procedure volume as predictors of subsequent hospital performance. Ann Surg 2006;243(3):411–7.

41. Birkmeyer JD, Siewers AE, Finlayson EV, et al. Hospital volume and surgical mortality in the United States. N Engl J Med 2002;346(15):1128–37.

42. Birkmeyer JD, Stukel TA, Siewers AE, et al. Surgeon volume and operative mortality in the United States. N Engl J Med 2003;349(22):2117–27.

43. Ghaferi AA, Birkmeyer JD, Dimick JB. Hospital volume and failure to rescue with high-risk surgery. Med Care 2011;49(12):1076–81.

44. Birkmeyer JD, Finks JF, O'Reilly A, et al. Surgical skill and complication rates after bariatric surgery. N Engl J Med 2013;369(15):1434–42.

45. Boudourakis LD, Wang TS, Roman SA, et al. Evolution of the surgeon-volume, patient-outcome relationship. Ann Surg 2009;250(1):159–65.

46. Halm EA, Lee C, Chassin MR. Is volume related to outcome in health care? A systematic review and methodologic critique of the literature. Ann Intern Med 2002;137(6):511–20.

47. Katz JN, Barrett J, Mahomed NN, et al. Association between hospital and surgeon procedure volume and the outcomes of total knee replacement. J Bone Joint Surg Am 2004;86(9):1909–16.

48. Losina E, Barrett J, Mahomed NN, et al. Early failures of total hip replacement: effect of surgeon volume. Arthritis Rheum 2004;50(4):1338–43.

49. Yao SL, Lu-Yao G. Population-based study of relationships between hospital volume of prostatectomies, patient outcomes, and length of hospital stay. J Natl Cancer Inst 1999;91(22):1950–6.

50. Tanna N, Clayton JL, Roostaeian J, et al. The volume-outcome relationship for immediate breast reconstruction. Plast Reconstr Surg 2012;129(1):19–24.

51. Cohen ME, Ko CY, Bilimoria KY, et al. Optimizing ACS NSQIP modeling for evaluation of surgical quality and risk: patient risk adjustment, procedure mix adjustment, shrinkage adjustment, and surgical focus. J Am Coll Surg 2013;217(2):336–46.e1.

52. Daley J, Khuri SF, Henderson W, et al. Risk adjustment of the postoperative morbidity rate for the comparative assessment of the quality of surgical care: results of the National Veterans Affairs Surgical Risk Study. J Am Coll Surg 1997;185(4):328–40.

53. Dimick JB, Osborne NH, Hall BL, et al. Risk adjustment for comparing hospital quality with surgery: how many variables are needed? J Am Coll Surg 2010;210(4):503–8.

54. Khuri SF, Daley J, Henderson W, et al. Risk adjustment of the postoperative mortality rate for the comparative assessment of the quality of surgical care: results of the National Veterans Affairs Surgical Risk Study. J Am Coll Surg 1997;185(4):315–27.

55. Dimick JB, Ghaferi AA, Osborne NH, et al. Reliability adjustment for reporting hospital outcomes with surgery. Ann Surg 2012;255(4):703–7.

56. Dimick JB, Staiger DO, Hall BL, et al. Composite measures for profiling hospitals on surgical morbidity. Ann Surg 2013;257(1):67–72.

57. O'Brien SM, Shahian DM, DeLong ER, et al. Quality measurement in adult cardiac surgery: part 2–Statistical considerations in composite measure scoring and provider rating. Ann Thorac Surg 2007;83(Suppl 4):S13–26.

58. Shahian DM, O'Brien SM, Normand SL, et al. Association of hospital coronary artery bypass volume with processes of care, mortality, morbidity, and the Society of Thoracic Surgeons composite quality score. J Thorac Cardiovasc Surg 2010;139(2):273–82.

59. Dimick JB, Birkmeyer NJ, Finks JF, et al. Composite measures for profiling hospitals on bariatric surgery performance. JAMA Surg 2014;149(1):10–6.

60. Bourne RB, Chesworth BM, Davis AM, et al. Patient satisfaction after total knee arthroplasty: who is satisfied and who is not? Clin Orthop Relat Res 2010;468(1):57–63.

61. Waljee JF, Chung KC. Objective functional outcomes and patient satisfaction after silicone metacarpophalangeal arthroplasty for rheumatoid arthritis. J Hand Surg Am 2012;37(1):47–54.

62. Hildon Z, Neuburger J, Allwood D, et al. Clinicians' and patients' views of metrics of change derived from patient reported outcome measures (PROMs) for comparing providers' performance of surgery. BMC Health Serv Res 2012;12:171.

63. Gutacker N, Bojke C, Daidone S, et al. Hospital variation in patient-reported outcomes at the level of EQ-5D dimensions: evidence from England. Med Decis Making 2013;33(6):804–18.

64. Parkin D, Devlin NJ. Using health status to measure NHS performance: casting light in dark places. BMJ Qual Saf 2012;21(4):355–6.

65. Devlin NJ, Parkin D, Browne J. Patient-reported outcome measures in the NHS: new methods for analysing and reporting EQ-5D data. Health Econ 2010;19(8):886–905.

66. Gutacker N, Bojke C, Daidone S, et al. Truly ineffi-cient or providing better quality of care? Analysing the relationship between risk-adjusted hospital costs and patients' health outcomes. Health Econ 2013;22(8):931–47.

67. Appleby J, Poteliakhoff E, Shah K, et al. Using patient-reported outcome measures to estimate cost-effectiveness of hip replacements in English hospitals. J R Soc Med 2013;106(8):323–31.

68. Coronini-Cronberg S, Appleby J, Thompson J. Application of patient-reported outcome measures (PROMs) data to estimate cost-effectiveness of hernia surgery in England. J R Soc Med 2013; 106(7):278–87.

69. Neuburger J, Hutchings A, van der Meulen J, et al. Using patient-reported outcomes (PROs) to compare the providers of surgery: does the choice of measure matter? Med Care 2013;51(6):517–23.

70. Hildon Z, Allwood D, Black N. Patients' and clini-cians' views of comparing the performance of pro-viders of surgery: a qualitative study. Health Expect 2012. [Epub ahead of print].

71. O'Connor AM, Llewellyn-Thomas HA, Flood AB. Modifying unwarranted variations in health care: shared decision making using patient decision AIDS. Health Aff (Millwood) 2004;(Suppl Variation): VAR63–72.

72. Scuffham PA, Ratcliffe J, Kendall E, et al. Engaging the public in healthcare decision-making: quanti-fying preferences for healthcare through citizens' juries. BMJ Open 2014;4(5):e005437.

73. Katz SJ, Lantz PM, Janz NK, et al. Patient involve-ment in surgery treatment decisions for breast can-cer. J Clin Oncol 2005;23(24):5526–33.

74. Fagerlin A, Lakhani I, Lantz PM, et al. An informed decision? Breast cancer patients and their knowl-edge about treatment. Patient Educ Couns 2006; 64(1–3):303–12.

75. Hawley ST, Lantz PM, Janz NK, et al. Factors asso-ciated with patient involvement in surgical treat-ment decision making for breast cancer. Patient Educ Couns 2007;65(3):387–95.

76. Lantz PM, Mujahid M, Schwartz K, et al. The influ-ence of race, ethnicity, and individual socioeco-nomic factors on breast cancer stage at diagnosis. Am J Public Health 2006;96(12):2173–8.

77. Truog RD. Patients and doctors–evolution of a rela-tionship. N Engl J Med 2012;366(7):581–5.

78. Sepucha KR, Fowler FJ Jr, Mulley AG Jr. Policy support for patient-centered care: the need for measurable improvements in decision quality. Health Aff (Millwood) 2004;(Suppl Variation): VAR54–62.

79. O'Connor AM, Rostom A, Fiset V, et al. Decision aids for patients facing health treatment or screening decisions: systematic review. BMJ 1999;319(7212):731–4.

80. O'Connor AM, Stacey D, Rovner D, et al. Decision aids for people facing health treatment or screening decisions. Cochrane Database Syst Rev 2001;(3):CD001431.

81. Schwartz LM, Woloshin S, Welch HG. Can patients interpret health information? An assessment of the medical data interpretation test. Med Decis Making 2005;25(3):290–300.

82. Bilimoria KY, Liu Y, Paruch JL, et al. Development and evaluation of the universal ACS NSQIP surgi-cal risk calculator: a decision aid and informed consent tool for patients and surgeons. J Am Coll Surg 2013;217(5):833–42.e1–3.

83. Waljee JF, Rogers MA, Alderman AK. Decision aids and breast cancer: do they influence choice for surgery and knowledge of treatment options? J Clin Oncol 2007;25(9):1067–73.

84. Post S, Selles R, McGrouther D, et al. Levels of ev-idence and quality of randomized controlled trials in hand and wrist surgery: an analysis of two major hand surgery journals. J Hand Surg Eur 2013. [Epub ahead of print].

85. Ahn C, Li R, Ahn B, et al. Hand and wrist research productivity in journals with high impact factors: a 20 year analysis. J Hand Surg Eur Vol 2012;37(3): 275–83.

86. Wright JG, Swiontkowski MF, Heckman JD. Intro-ducing levels of evidence to the journal. J Bone Joint Surg Am 2003;85(1):1–3.

87. Hentz RV, Meals RA, Stern P, et al. Levels of Evi-dence and the Journal of Hand Surgery. J Hand Surg Am 2005;30(5):891–2.

88. Sackett DL, Rosenberg WM, Gray J, et al. Evi-dence based medicine: what it is and what it isn't. BMJ 1996;312(7023):71–2.

89. Murphy MM, Simons JP, Hill JS, et al. Pancreatic resection: a key component to reducing racial dis-parities in pancreatic adenocarcinoma. Cancer 2009;115(17):3979–90.

90. Regenbogen SE, Gawande AA, Lipsitz SR, et al. Do differences in hospital and surgeon quality explain racial disparities in lower-extremity vascular ampu-tations? Ann Surg 2009;250(3):424–31.

91. Newacheck PW, Hung YY, Park MJ, et al. Dispar-ities in adolescent health and health care: does so-cioeconomic status matter? Health Serv Res 2003; 38(5):1235–52.

92. Grewal R, MacDermid JC, King GJ, et al. Open reduction internal fixation versus percutaneous pinning with external fixation of distal radius frac-tures: a prospective, randomized clinical trial. J Hand Surg Am 2011;36(12):1899–906.

93. Zollinger PE, Tuinebreijer WE, Breederveld RS, et al. Can vitamin C prevent complex regional pain syndrome in patients with wrist fractures? A random-ized, controlled, multicenter dose-response study. J Bone Joint Surg Am 2007;89(7):1424–31.

94. Dimick JB, Nicholas LH, Ryan AM, et al. Bariatric surgery complications before vs after implementation of a national policy restricting coverage to centers of excellence. JAMA 2013;309(8):792–9.

95. Chen NC, Shauver MJ, Chung KC. Cost-effectiveness of open partial fasciectomy, needle aponeurotomy, and collagenase injection for dupuytren contracture. J Hand Surg Am 2011; 36(11):1826–34.e2.

96. Shauver MJ, Yin H, Banerjee M, et al. Current and future national costs to medicare for the treatment of distal radius fracture in the elderly. J Hand Surg Am 2011;36(8):1282–7.

97. Alderman AK, Wei Y, Birkmeyer JD. Use of breast reconstruction after mastectomy following the Women's Health and Cancer Rights Act. JAMA 2006;295(4):387–8.

98. Giladi AM, Aliu O, Chung KC. The effect of medicaid expansion in new york state on use of subspecialty surgical procedures by medicaid beneficiaries and the uninsured. J Am Coll Surg 2014;218(5):889–97.

Evidence-Based Medicine in Hand Surgery
Clinical Applications and Future Direction

Brian Zafonte, MD, PhD, Robert M. Szabo, MD, MPH*

KEYWORDS

- Evidence-based medicine • Hand surgery • Upper extremity surgery

KEY POINTS

- Level 1 evidence has unified patient care strategies for many common hand and upper extremity problems.
- There are pathologies for which our current evidence base has not yet unified the "best" treatment, and in some cases the management remains controversial.
- For rare, heterogeneous, and atypical clinical presentations, data from level 4 studies are often more helpful in guiding treatment.

AREAS OF HAND AND UPPER EXTREMITY SURGERY WHERE EBM SHOULD UNIFY TREATMENT STRATEGIES
The Treatment of Lateral Epicondylitis

Corticosteroid injections are ubiquitously used in the management of lateral epicondylitis. They are relatively easy to administer by physicians, often requested by patients, and their safety profile is well established. However, their broad use in treating lateral epicondylitis is not data driven, especially given the noninflammatory pathogenesis of the disease. Multiple prospective randomized controlled studies have evaluated corticosteroid injections in comparison with placebo,[1–3] observation,[4] physical therapy,[5] or their combinations.[6,7] The results demonstrate that corticosteroids are generally effective in the short term (~6 weeks), but no long-term benefit (>1–2 years) is found, particularly with regard to pain, grip strength, and Disabilities of Arm, Shoulder, and Hand (DASH) score. Meta-analyses also have failed to demonstrate a favorable long-term advantage of using corticosteroid injections for lateral epicondylitis.[8–10] In addition, studies comparing different corticosteroid formulations[8,11] (eg, triamcinolone vs methylprednisolone vs betamethasone, vs dexamethasone vs hydrocortisone), number[12,13] and frequency[8,14] of injections, or site of injection/injection technique[7,8,15,16] have also not proven any long-term benefit over placebo or watchful waiting. With respect to evaluating corticosteroid versus plasma-rich protein (PRP) injections, 3 recent level 1 studies have found differing results.[17–19] The results from Krogh and colleagues[17] favored PRP at 1 month but were no different at 3 months. In contrast, at the 1-year and 2-year follow-up, Peerbooms and colleagues[19] and Gosens and colleagues[18] demonstrated that patients treated with PRP had significantly better DASH and Visual Analog Scale (VAS) scores. However, all patients in these 2 studies significantly improved over baseline, and neither study included a placebo or observation-only group, so it is difficult to draw definitive conclusions about the efficacy of PRP for lateral epicondylitis.

Other studies examining the utility of newer treatment modalities for lateral epicondylitis have

Disclosures: None.
Department of Orthopaedic Surgery, University of California, 4860 Y Street, Suite 3800, Davis, Sacramento, CA 95817, USA
* Corresponding author.
E-mail address: rmszabo@ucdavis.edu

Hand Clin 30 (2014) 269–283
http://dx.doi.org/10.1016/j.hcl.2014.04.005

been reported, including prolotherapy,[20] autologous blood injections,[21,22] acupuncture,[23] extracorporeal shock wave therapy,[24] and Botox injections.[15] Although there is interest and innovation in these "newer" treatments, none of these modalities have demonstrated any statistically significant long-term favorable outcome. Additional research is ongoing to examine if any will emerge better than the natural self-limited course of the disease.

EBM bottom line recommendation
No routine corticosteroid injections for lateral epicondylitis.

The Use of Antibiotics During Elective Hand Surgery

Although antibiotics are broadly used in hand and upper-extremity surgery requiring deep dissection, bone reconstruction, and the use of implants, their utility in elective hand surgery is much less established, particularly for those operations lasting less than 2 hours. The emergence of drug-resistant bacteria and other antibiotic-related complications is forcing the surgical community to reevaluate the prolific use of intraoperative antibiotics. Now there is strong evidence against the routine use of prophylactic antibiotics during elective hand surgery. Most of these studies have centered on carpal tunnel release (CTR) surgery. Hanssen and colleagues'[25] large retrospective review of 3620 carpal tunnel release surgeries reported an infection rate of 0.47%, which is consistent with previous reports in the literature. Although they did not formally evaluate the effect of prophylactic antibiotics on surgical site infection, 80% of their patients received no intraoperative antibiotics. Moreover, Harness and colleagues[26] performed a multicenter retrospective review examining the correlation between antibiotic use and the development of a postoperative surgical site infection in 3003 patients. They found no statistical difference in infection rates between patients who received prophylactic antibiotics and those who did not, including a subanalysis of diabetic and nondiabetic cohorts. Kleinert and colleagues[27] also found no evidence that the use of prophylactic antibiotics in carpal tunnel surgery was predictive of infection.

Data have also emerged for soft tissue hand surgery cases other than carpal tunnel release. In their retrospective review of 600 patients, Tosti and colleagues[28] studied infection rates in patients undergoing trigger finger release, soft tissue mass excision, and first dorsal compartment release, in addition to CTR. Their patients manifested only superficial infections and the overall infection rate was 0.66%. Patients who received antibiotics had an infection rate of 0.47%, whereas the infection rate in those who received no antibiotics was 0.77%. These rates were not statistically significant. In a prospective randomized study of 1340 patients, Aydin and colleagues[29] divided patients into 4 groups based on the depth and type of surgery. Group 1 included surgery limited to the skin and subcutaneous tissue, whereas group 2 involved surgery to tendons, nerves, and arteries. Group 3 included surgeries involving bone and joints, and group 4 included patients who had skin-loss defects. Half of the patients in each group received prophylactic antibiotics, and the researchers compared infection rates between those patients who received intraoperative antibiotics and those who received no antibiotics. They found no statistical differences in infection rates between antibiotic use versus placebo in any of the 4 groups. In another large retrospective review of 8850 outpatient hand surgery cases, Bykowski and colleagues[30] examine the rate of surgical site infection with the use of antibiotics. Infection rates were not statistically different between those patients who received antibiotics and those who received none. In addition, their subgroup analysis of those patients who were more high risk for infection (those with diabetes and those who smoke) also failed to demonstrate that antibiotics reduce surgical site infections.

These studies demonstrate that the routine use of prophylactic antibiotics in elective soft tissue hand surgery less than 2 hours long is not warranted. Despite this evidence, some hospital systems continue to mandate the continued routine use of prophylactic antibiotics. Future directions should include work in this area by researchers and administrators alike to create guidelines that promote evidence-based, safe, and effective antibiotic use in upper extremity surgery.

EBM bottom line recommendation
No routine prophylactic antibiotics for elective soft tissue hand surgery cases lasting less than 2 hours.

The Repair of Zone II Flexor Tendon Injuries

There is no shortage of literature describing repair of zone II flexor tendon injuries with regard to technique and suture type and configuration. There is strong consensus that surgical repair is not warranted for incomplete tendon injuries involving less than 60% of the cross-sectional area, especially if finger range of motion is not impeded. However, tendon disruptions greater than 60% should be repaired. The ideal repair should be strong enough to withstand early active hand therapy protocols to minimize the risk of tendon re-rupture. Some investigators have suggested this minimum strength should be 73.5 N.[31,32] Many biomechanical studies have demonstrated that increasing the number of core sutures directly increases the strength of the repair.[33–39] Two-strand core repairs have a range of 28.0 to 33.9 N of ultimate strength before failure, whereas 4-strand and 6-strand repairs have ranges of 40.7 to 80.0 N and 53.6 to 78.7 N, respectively. The variations in strength seen in this in vitro data are likely due to the different suture materials and techniques used. Other biomechanical work has shown that the use of epitendinous sutures, dorsal placement of core sutures, and the use of locking sutures all increase strength of the repair,[40–43] but clinical comparative outcome studies are lacking. Many studies using a specific repair technique have patient outcome data, but there are only 2 reports that directly compare different suture techniques in patients with zone II injuries. One study compared a 6-strand Lin/Tsai repair technique to a 2-strand modified Kessler technique. The 6-strand repair group had a statistically significant better range of motion and a lower complication rate.[44] Those patients also had a lower re-rupture rate, but that result was not significant. The rehabilitation protocols were not standardized between the 2 groups, thereby likely confounding the effects of the suture repair. In the other study, Osada and colleagues[45] compared 2 different 6-strand repairs and reported a 96% excellent result based on the original Strickland criterion. There were no clinically significant differences in the outcomes of the 2 groups after average follow-up of 13 months (range 6–51 months), and there were no tendon ruptures in either group.

Many types and sizes of suture material are available for flexor tendon repairs, and crucially, the suture material must be strong and slender to avoid weak, bulky repairs. It must also not promote scar formation or foreign body reaction. Most surgeons use a 3-0 or 4-0 nonabsorbable polyfilament because of their better gliding properties and similar tensile strength compared with stainless steel sutures,[32] and these repairs have been shown to withstand early postoperative motion therapy.[33] Absorbable sutures are not used because they stimulate a significant local tissue reaction with subsequent adhesion formation,[46] even though the results of one retrospective study showed comparable clinical outcomes versus using nonabsorbable suture material.[47] The TenoFix (Ortheon Medical, Winter Park, FL, USA) device demonstrated similar repair strength and good clinical outcomes compared with standard 3-0 and 4-0 sutures in biomechanical and clinical studies[48–51]; however, its use is often limited by inadequate tendon exposure or tendon injuries that preclude the placement of both suture anchors. Last, although monofilaments have better knot-tying capabilities, they are not as strong as braided sutures and thus they are most commonly used only as epitendinous sutures.

Future directions, as surgeons continue to develop new strategies that promote early active range of motion and function without sacrificing the integrity of the repair, should be directed at providing high-level clinical evidence studies instead of more cadaver biomechanical studies.

EBM bottom line recommendation
Use a nonabsorbable polyfilament suture with a minimum of 4-strand core suture technique with an epitendinous suture and initiate a postoperative passive or active motion therapy protocol.

Postoperative Splinting After Carpal Tunnel Release

Carpal tunnel syndrome (CTS) is the most common compressive neuropathy encountered, and open carpal tunnel release (CTR) is the gold standard treatment. Not surprisingly, a multitude of postoperative CTR regimens exists and vary from surgeon to surgeon. Whether or not to perform postoperative immobilization has been an area of interest and multiple randomized level 1 studies have been undertaken to address that question. Collectively, they have shown that splinting after CTR is not advantageous. Bhatia and colleagues,[52] Bury and colleagues,[53] and Finsen and colleagues[54] treated patients after CTR with plaster splint immobilization for 48 hours, 2 weeks, and 4 weeks, respectively. They found no differences with respect to pain, range of motion, strength, or time to return to work between patients who were immobilized and those who received no splinting. Huemer and colleagues[55] repeated electrical studies 3 months after CTR and found no statistically significant difference in distal motor latency between patients who were splinted and those who had no immobilization. In a study by Cook and colleagues,[56] patients were randomized to 2 weeks of splinting versus an immediate motion protocol. Subjects were evaluated at 2 weeks, 1 month, and 3 and 6 months. The non-splinted group showed faster return to normal activities, earlier return to employment, and quicker recovery of grip and key pinch strength. Moreover, patients in the splinted wrist group had increased pain and scar tenderness in the first month after surgery. These findings suggested that splinting the wrist after CTR can be harmful.

In 2008 Henry and colleagues[57] reported on the practice of postoperative splinting after CTR among members of the American Society for Surgery of the Hand. They used a questionnaire to ascertain if and for how long patients were splinted after CTR; 53% of respondents (n = 1091) reported using full-time splinting postoperatively, and the most common duration of immobilization was 7 days (range 1–42 days). This trend was consistent among all hand surgeons irrespective of their background training in orthopedic, plastic, or general surgery. In addition to full-time splinting after CTR, a small percentage of surgeons used a period of night splinting (5%), whereas 1% of surgeons used only night splinting postoperatively. The good news from this study was that the 53% prevalence rate of splinting after CTR was actually a downward trend when compared with past surveys conducted 10 and 20 years earlier (82% in 1987[58] and 69% in 1997[59]). In 2009, after reviewing the data, the American Academy of Orthopedic Surgeons (AAOS) issued clinical practice guidelines for CTS recommending that the wrist not be immobilized postoperatively after routine carpal tunnel surgery.[60]

So while postoperative splinting after CTR may have been initially recommended to prevent tendon bowstringing and median nerve scarring, these complications are rarely encountered and, moreover, there is good evidence to argue against the practice of routine postoperative splinting after CTR.

EBM bottom line recommendation
No routine postoperative immobilization after carpal tunnel release.

The Surgical Treatment of Cubital Tunnel Syndrome

Cubital tunnel syndrome is the second most commonly seen compressive neuropathy, and its treatment encompasses a variety of surgical procedures. The 2 most commonly performed surgical techniques are simple decompression and anterior transposition of the ulnar nerve with either subcutaneous or submuscular placement. Many studies have been performed to compare these modalities in an effort to identify the one treatment that yields clinically superior results. Gervasio and colleagues,[61] in a level 1 randomized study, compared simple decompression to anterior submuscular transposition of the ulnar nerve. They included 35 patients (all Dellon stage 3) in each group and evaluated all patients at 6 months after surgery by using the Bishop rating system. They found no statistically significant differences in any of the outcome measures between the

2 groups. In a similar study by Biggs and Curtis,[62] no clinical differences were found at 1 month, 6 months, or 1 year postoperatively, although submuscular transposition was associated with a higher incidence of significant wound complications. In addition, Bartels and colleagues[63] compared simple decompression with anterior subcutaneous transposition in 150 patients split into 2 groups. The primary measure was clinical outcome 1 year after surgery: 65% of patients who underwent simple decompression and 70% of patients who underwent anterior subcutaneous transposition achieved excellent or good results, which was not significantly different. However, the complication rate was statistically lower in the simple decompression group (9.6% vs 31.1%). Because of equivalent outcomes with lower complication rates, the investigators advised performing simple decompression, even in the presence of ulnar nerve subluxation.

Meta-analyses of level 1 studies evaluating simple ulnar nerve decompression versus transposition have yielded similar findings. In one meta-analysis of 10 studies involving 449 simple decompressions, 342 subcutaneous transpositions, and 115 submuscular transpositions, there was no statistically significant clinical difference between the groups.[64] Further subanalyses on the basis of transposition technique also failed to identify any clinically significant outcome. A second meta-analysis of 5 level 1 studies including 361 patients compared simple decompression to subcutaneous and submuscular transposition. The results again demonstrated equivalent clinical outcomes.[65] No significant study heterogeneity was found within these meta-analyses.

The treatment of cubital tunnel syndrome continues to evolve, especially as there remains no consensus as to the superiority of one particular surgical technique. Although several surgical modalities yield equivalent clinical outcomes, the current evidence demonstrates that simple ulnar nerve decompression is the least invasive technique associated with the smallest amount of surgical complications.

EBM bottom line recommendation
Perform simple ulnar nerve decompression for routine proximal ulnar nerve compression.

WHERE STRONG EVIDENCE HAS STILL FAILED TO UNIFY CONSENSUS ON TREATMENT
Thumb Basilar Joint Arthritis

Osteoarthritis at the base of the thumb causes severe pain and deformity, and results in significant patient disability. More than 15 different surgical methods have been described with the goals of relieving pain while promoting stability, motion, and strength recovery. Although there is great interest in identifying the optimal surgical procedure, no one technique has emerged superior to the rest, particularly with respect to pain, physical function, and global patient well-being.

In 2004, Martou and colleagues[66] published their systemic review that examined 8 reviews and 18 comparative technique studies with the goal to identify the "best" surgical technique for treating thumb basilar joint arthritis. The techniques included in their analysis were trapeziectomy with and without interposition, arthrodesis, osteotomy, and joint replacement. They found great variability in outcome measures and no specific technique was identified to provide superior results. In looking specifically at the comparative study data, ligament reconstruction and tendon interposition (LRTI) had no additional benefit when compared with carpometacarpal (CMC) fusion and trapeziectomy alone or with tendon interposition.

The Cochrane group has investigated studies on different surgical methods for treating thumb basilar joint arthritis. Wajon and colleagues[67] in 2005 examined level 1 randomized trials and concluded that no procedure was superior over another. Interestingly, they found that those patients who had trapeziectomy alone had fewer complications overall, whereas those who had LRTI had more complications, including scar tenderness, tendon adhesion or rupture, sensory changes, or type 1 complex regional pain syndrome. The Cochrane group updated their review in 2009 and at that time one additional procedure had been described, the Artelon joint resurfacing, which was included in the analysis. Again Wajon and colleagues[68] concluded that no single procedure produces greater benefit over the other surgical options, but trapeziectomy alone was associated with fewer complications than trapeziectomy with LRTI.

A recent review by Vermeulen and colleagues[69] in 2011 compared the 8 most commonly used surgical techniques (volar ligament reconstruction, metacarpal osteotomy, CMC fusion, joint replacement, trapeziectomy, trapeziectomy with tendon interposition, trapeziectomy with ligament reconstruction, and trapeziectomy with LRTI). Their results are in agreement with previous work that has failed to identify any one particular surgical technique as superior to the rest. Moreover, it was again found that trapeziectomy with LRTI was associated with a higher complication rate versus performing trapeziectomy alone. However, the relatively short follow-up in these studies

(~1 year) precludes the assessment of long-term outcome comparisons.

Although multiple types of suspension and implant arthroplasty in combination with trapeziectomy have been described with good outcomes, recent studies have advocated performing trapeziectomy alone. Davis and Pace[70] undertook a randomized prospective study of 113 patients split into 2 groups and compared trapeziectomy alone with trapeziectomy with LRTI. They assessed the patients at 3 months and 1 year and found no statistically significant differences in grip strength, DASH score, or Patient Evaluation Measure outcome score. Gray and Meals[71] also reported on the outcome of trapeziectomy with hematoma distraction in their series. At 6.5 years follow-up, 18 of 22 patients were pain free, had good range of motion, and showed an average of 21% and 11% increases in grip and pinch strength, respectively. The outcomes from trapeziectomy alone have proven that it is a safe and effective procedure, yet surgeons still incorporate with it other arthroplasty techniques. Because long-term (>1 year) data from level 1 comparative studies are lacking, it seems many surgeons are still convinced of the possible long-term benefit of other surgeries, particularly trapeziectomy with LRTI. The persistent popularity of performing trapeziectomy with LRTI was demonstrated in a 2012 survey of hand surgeons. Wolf and colleagues[72] queried members of the American Society for Surgery of the Hand to evaluate current trends in the management of thumb CMC arthritis. They found that 62% of 1156 respondents prefer trapeziectomy with LTRI as their treatment of choice for Eaton stage III arthritis. In addition, nearly half of respondents indicated that trapeziectomy with LRTI was their preferred method for treating scaphotrapeziotrapezoidal arthritis.

It is clear that our surgical management of thumb basilar joint arthritis continues to evolve. As more robust studies on CMC fusion and joint replacement are done, and additional level 1 data emerge on long-term outcomes, the future evidence should enable hand surgeons to reach consensus on the best available surgical technique.

EBM bottom line recommendation
Short-term evidence suggests removal of the trapezium alone is the preferred surgical treatment of thumb basilar joint arthritis.

Pronator Quadratus Repair After Distal Radius Surgery

Whether or not to repair the pronator quadratus (PQ) in the treatment of distal radius fractures with volar plating is an active area of interest among wrist surgeons. Proponents of PQ repair cite restoration of pronation strength, protection of flexor tendons, and stabilization of the distal radio-ulnar joint as benefits. Often the muscle tissue sustains trauma from the injury, which prevents repair, and assessing the integrity of the repair postoperatively is difficult. It is also possible that overtightening of the PQ repair could cause decreased forearm rotation. Currently, the impact of PQ repair on clinical outcome remains undefined.

Hershman and colleagues[73] retrospectively examined 112 patients with orthopaedic trauma association types 23-A through 23-C distal radius fractures that were treated with open reduction and internal fixation (ORIF) with volar plating. Half of the patients underwent PQ repair. The primary outcome measure was forearm range of motion and they evaluated patients at 6 weeks and 3, 6, and 12 months after surgery. They found no difference in pronation between the 2 groups. Their secondary outcome measures for grip strength, pain levels, DASH scores, and complications were also similar. They did, however, demonstrate a statistically significant improvement in radial deviation in the group without PQ repair. Ahsan and Yao[74] found similar results in their retrospective study comparing complete versus incomplete PQ repair during volar plating of distal radius fractures. Two prospective level II studies also have shown no clinical benefit to repairing the PQ during volar plating of distal radius fractures. Swigart and colleagues[75] graded the extent of the PQ injury at the time of surgery and found no correlation between the extent of injury and postoperative outcomes. In addition, by placing trackable radiopaque hemoclips along the PQ repair interface, they demonstrated only 1 failure at the 3-month follow-up. They concluded that whereas PQ repairs are generally durable, repairing the muscle does not offer any significant motion or strength advantage over not performing PQ repair. The recent work by Tosti and Ilyas[76] support these earlier finding as well. At follow-up of 1 year there were no statistically significant differences in range of motion, grip strength, and DASH and VAS scores between patients who had PQ repair and those who did not undergo PQ repair.

Even though 83% of hand surgeons reported routinely attempting a PQ repair after distal radius fixation,[75] the current evidence seems to indicate that PQ repair may not be necessary. However, this conclusion is based on retrospective and level II studies and the question as to the effect on tendon irritation and rupture related to repair or no-repair has not been investigated. Future directions should be aimed at obtaining data from randomized clinical trials to further answer these questions.

EBM bottom line recommendation
It is surgeon preference as to whether or not to repair the PQ after volar plating of distal radius fractures.

Open Versus Endoscopic Surgery for Carpal Tunnel Release

Endoscopic carpal tunnel release (ECTR) has gained in popularity over the years, but open carpal tunnel release (OCTR) remains the gold standard treatment for patients with CTS. Many studies have compared ECTR with OCTR in an effort to assess the benefit of ECTR. The most recent Cochrane Collaboration on the subject was reported in 2007. In that report, Scholten and colleagues[77] examined the evidence from 16 level 1 studies that compared the efficacy of ECTR to OCTR. They found that ECTR did not provide significantly better relief of symptoms when compared with OCTR, and this included both short-term and long-term follow-up data. However, some of these studies indicated that patients undergoing ECTR were able to return to work or activities of daily living (ADLs) earlier than those receiving OCRT. That conclusion also was reported in a meta-analysis of 3 studies involving 294 patients, where it was demonstrated that ECTR resulted in, on average, a 6-day earlier return to work (range 3–9 days) or ADLs.[78–80] No major complications were reported in either of the 2 groups. The investigators concluded that OCTR should remain the standard of care.

The AAOS physician work group published clinical diagnosis and treatment guidelines for CTS in 2008.[81] Part of the report was aimed at comparing ECTR to OCTR. Their review showed that ECTR was favored for outcome measures of pain at 12 weeks' duration until return to work, pinch strength at 12 weeks, and wound complications. OCTR was preferred with respect to the complication of reversible nerve damage, which is seen more with ECTR. At 1-year post CTR, there were no significant differences in any outcome measure. In looking at comparative outcomes at 5 years after CTR, Atroshi and colleagues[82] compared CTS symptom severity and CTS functional status scores between the ECTR and OCTR groups, and found no statistical difference.

Overall, there is no clear evidence that ECTR is superior to OCTR. Although the evidence may show questionable differences in the early postoperative period, long-term outcomes are equivalent. In addition, many surgeons would argue that the patient morbidity and subsequent health care burden from an ECTR-induced median nerve injury far outweighs any short-term benefit conferred by ECTR. Therefore, OCTR remains the gold standard treatment.

EBM bottom line recommendation
  OCTR is still the preferred method of treatment for CTS, but ECTR is an acceptable alternative.

Steroid Injections into the Carpal Tunnel

Local corticosteroid injections are a common practice in the nonsurgical management of symptomatic patients with CTS. Steroid injections are relatively safe, quick, and easy to perform, and patients may experience speedy relief of symptoms. Many studies have been undertaken to assess the efficacy of corticosteroid injections for patients with CTS. Two level 1 randomized controlled trials demonstrated significant clinical improvement of CTS symptoms within 1 month compared with placebo. In the first study, Dammers and colleagues[83] injected methylprednisolone proximal to the carpal tunnel and found that 77% of patients had no symptoms at 1 month follow-up. Moreover, at 1 year, 50% of those patients remained symptom free. Later, Armstrong and colleagues[84] performed betamethasone injections and found similar results; 70% of their patients achieved relief of symptoms, and these patients also showed improvement on their electrical studies and subjective outcome scores. These data demonstrate that corticosteroid injections are effective in the short-term for managing symptomatic CTS. In examining midterm effects of corticosteroid injections, Visser and colleagues[85] reported 63% symptom relief at 6 months, 48% relief at 12 months, and 34% relief at 18 months. In the same study, the investigators correlated the severity of electrodiagnostic testing with outcome and found that patients with mild CTS had the best results at 15 months (50% symptom-free).

In a study assessing the number of injections given, performing 2 local corticosteroid injections versus 1 injection did not yield any further clinical improvement over performing 1 injection alone.[86] Studies characterizing site of injection (distal vs proximal),[87] dose and formulation of steroid,[88,89] and steroid half-life[89] have not shown significant findings. In diabetic patients, Catalano and colleagues[90] recently showed that corticosteroid injections do not significantly clinically affect glucose homeostasis. Studies have also been performed comparing the utility of local corticosteroid injections to other nonsurgical modalities, and the results seem to favor corticosteroid injections.

There is good evidence that corticosteroid injections for CTS are efficacious early on; however, achieving consistent and long-term relief has not been realized. Moreover, a recent study reported that the use of preoperative corticosteroid injections was associated with worse long-term outcomes after CTR. In their work, Vahi and colleagues[91] retrospectively collected data on subjective patient outcomes and the number of preoperative steroid injections patients received (majority receiving 1–3). They used regression modeling to analyze the relationship between the presence of postoperative symptoms and the number of preoperative steroid injections; 164 patients were included in the study and the follow-up was 5 to 6 years after CTR. They found that each additional injection after the index one was associated with small but significant increases in occurrence of pain, paresthesia, and nocturnal awakenings. It is clear that additional work is necessary to help us refine our indications and use profile for corticosteroid injections in the treatment of CTS.

EBM bottom line recommendation
  Corticosteroid injection into the carpal tunnel is an effective short-term treatment for patients with CTS.

The Utility of Platelet-Rich Plasma

Platelet-rich plasma (PRP) has been introduced as a possible new therapy in the treatment of tendinopathy and tendon injury. Two areas of active research for PRP in hand surgery are the management of lateral elbow epicondylitis and flexor tendon injuries. Early in vitro data demonstrated the ability of PRP to stimulate cellular proliferation and collagen production in human tenocyte cultures.[92] Morizaki and colleagues[93] looked at the effects of PRP on bone marrow stromal cell transplants in tendon healing. Using an in vitro canine tendon-healing model, they found that PRP significantly increased the strength and stiffness of healing tendons compared with control and bone marrow stromal cell only groups. Bosch and colleagues[94] reported similar results in an in vivo equine model. Their data showed that an intratendinous PRP injection enhanced the quality of digital flexor tendon repairs. The PRP group was found to have increased collagen, glycosaminoglycan, and DNA content. These tendons also showed a higher elastic modulus and strength at failure. Sato and colleagues[95] recently published comparable results using a rabbit model. These initial animal studies indicate that PRP may have the potential to enhance flexor tendon healing. However, it remains to be seen whether PRP will be shown to be relevant in human studies.

Because PRP has been shown to be a general stimulant in tendon repair, its utility also has been investigated for use in treating lateral elbow epicondylitis. Gosens and colleagues,[18] in a level 1 study, declared that patients treated with PRP had significantly better DASH and VAS scores at 2-year follow-up, compared with the corticosteroid group. Peerbooms and colleagues[19] reported the same findings at 1-year follow-up. In that study, all patients significantly improved over baseline, but there was no placebo group, so definitive conclusions on PRP efficacy can not be drawn.

An important aspect of using PRP in patient care is the cost factor. Most insurance companies either only partially cover or do not reimburse at all for incorporating PRP into treatment. At this point, there is no clear evidence that PRP is useful in human conditions, yet physicians have been quick to adopt this modality.

EBM bottom line recommendation
> *There is no strong evidence for the use of PRP in hand surgery. Its cost-effectiveness clearly shows that it should not be recommended at this time.*

Metacarpophalangeal Joint Arthroplasty in Rheumatoid Arthritis

With the advent of tumor necrosis factor-alpha inhibitors, the medical management of patients with rheumatoid arthritis (RA) has been transformed. Still, the operative treatment of the rheumatoid hand remains an area of active interest among hand surgeons, especially because hand function correlates with overall patient well-being. Implant arthroplasty has been the gold standard treatment for symptomatic metacarpophalangeal (MCP) deformities, and silicone arthroplasty is the most commonly performed procedure. Many studies have examined outcomes of silicone MCP arthroplasty. Waljee and Chung[96] reported on objective and subjective outcomes in 46 patients after silicone MCP arthroplasty. In their multicenter study, they followed patients for 2 years after surgery and evaluated subjective function using the Michigan Hand Outcome Questionnaire. They also analyzed grip and pinch strength, finger position, and MCP arc of motion. They found that patients who achieved improvement in extensor lag, ulnar drift, and MCP range of motion were satisfied with their treatment, despite only modest gains in pinch and grip strength. The same group has previously reported similar patient satisfaction rates using silicone MCP arthroplasty in patients with RA,[97–99] and others have published promising intermediate-term results.[100–103] However, long-term outcomes are not as promising. In a long-term follow-up study, Goldfarb and Stern[104] found that both subjective and objective outcomes decrease with time. At an average follow-up of 14 years (range 6–21 years), patients lost the immediate postoperative improvements in motion, extension deficit, and ulnar drift, although not all gains was lost compared with preoperative measures. Moreover, a significant percentage of the implants were either broken (63%) or deformed (22%) as well. In addition, only 38% of patients expressed satisfaction and only 27% of hands were pain-free at final follow-up.

These data suggest that silicone MCP arthroplasty in patients with RA yields good short-term results with high patient satisfaction. But improvements in hand function and cosmesis are lost in the long term. Therefore, selecting patients for surgery should be carefully considered and understanding patient expectations must be thoroughly discussed.

EBM bottom line recommendation
> *There is no strong evidence for or against silicone MCP arthroplasty in rheumatoid disease based on deformity.*

WHERE THE EBM JURY IS STILL OUT
Distal Radius Fractures: Cast Versus External Fixation Versus Open Reduction Internal Fixation

There are more than 2000 studies and reports on distal radius fractures in the literature; however, treatment in 2014 remains controversial. Traditionally, distal radius fractures were treated with casting, but surgical strategies have gained favor and are now widely used. But what does the evidence show? A plethora of studies, including those examining casting, closed reduction with percutaneous pinning, external fixation, and open reduction internal fixation (ORIF) with dorsal and volar plates have been published. Most of the ORIF studies have focused on volar distal radius plating, which has gained tremendous popularity in recent years. Despite the extensive data on the subject, treatment remains highly variable.

The Cochrane Collaboration has examined multiple options of distal radius fracture treatment. Their most recent report compared level 1 data on different methods of external fixation in adults.[105] Overall they found equivalent results with respect to function and deformity comparing bridging versus pins and plaster external fixation, nonbridging versus bridging fixation, using hydroxyapatite versus standard uncoated pins, and static versus dynamic external fixation. They concluded that the evidence was insufficient to identify a superior method of external fixation. The question of whether or not percutaneous pinning yields superior results versus conservative measures (eg, casting), was addressed in another Cochrane investigation. Handoll and colleagues[106] found that percutaneous pinning of unstable distal radius fractures was associated with improved outcomes in general, but a higher incidence of complications was seen using the Kapandji technique when different pinning methods were compared and when biodegradable pins were used compared with standard metal pins. They concluded that the role of percutaneous pinning in treating distal radius fractures remains to be fully characterized. A third Cochrane Collaboration report was aimed to identify the best type of surgical intervention for treating unstable distal radius fractures in adults. Handoll and Madhok[107] evaluated 48 trials involving 3371 patients with displaced, comminuted, and unstable distal radius fractures. The main patient cohorts were composed of older female patients and 50% of the trials compared surgery to cast immobilization. They found that surgery was associated with better bone alignment and restoration of radiological parameters after fractures healed, but the evidence was inconclusive in demonstrating that surgery produced better functional and clinical outcomes, nor was a superior surgical technique identified. These Cochrane reviews are based on level 1 studies and, in their inability to formulate definitive management strategies based on the data, illustrate the ongoing controversy, and frustration, regarding the optimal treatment of distal radius fractures among wrist surgeons.

Since the Cochrane studies were released, additional work has been published comparing surgical techniques, with particular emphasis on comparing volar plating with other methods of stabilization. In comparing locked volar plating versus external fixation, the cohort study by Wright and colleagues[108] found better radiological outcomes in the volar plate group, but equivalent DASH and Patient-Rated Wrist Evaluation (PRWE) scores. Jeudy and colleagues[109] performed a prospective randomized study on 75 patients split into 2 groups. They found that patients in the ORIF group achieved better articular reduction and clinical outcomes compared with patients who underwent external fixation, and patients in the external fixation group had more infections as well. In the past 2 years, at least 4 meta-analyses of level 1 data comparing volar plating with external fixation have been published.[110–113] These studies uniformly show higher DASH scores in the external fixation group.

However, there were better functional outcomes in the volar plating group in one study, improved function in the external fixation group in another study, and equivalent functional outcomes between the 2 groups in the third study. Consistently though, volar plating produced superior radiological outcomes in all studies. In their recent study comparing volar plating versus percutaneous pinning versus external fixation, Grewal and colleagues[114] were also unable to identify a superior method of surgical stabilization. They found that early subjective outcomes favored volar plating, but at 1 year, all scores equalized among the 3 groups. Collectively, the heterogeneity of results from these studies illustrate that additional work is needed to produce high-quality data that will unify treatment plans for distal radius fractures.

The Wrist and Radius Injury Surgery Trial (WRIST) was born out of a deficiency in the quality of evidence on distal radius fractures, and from inconclusive treatment guidelines from the AAOS. WRIST is a collaboration of 21 hand surgery centers that have launched a multicenter clinical trial aimed to compare percutaneous pinning versus external fixation versus ORIF with volar-locking plates in patients 60 years or older. This will be the largest trial on distal radius fractures to date, and the results from this initiative should help surgeons define and overcome barriers to unifying surgical stabilization methods in optimizing distal radius fracture care.

EBM bottom line recommendation
The optimal management of unstable distal radius fractures remains controversial with respect to cast immobilization versus surgery, and surgical technique.

Nondisplaced Scaphoid Fractures

Controversy continues to surround the optimal management of acute nondisplaced scaphoid fractures. Traditionally, these fractures were and are still treated with cast immobilization, but there has been a recent trend toward surgical fixation, particularly using percutaneous methods. Bedi and colleagues[115] reported very good results in their case series on ORIF of nondisplaced waist fractures using a limited dorsal approach with compression screw fixation. The researchers examined wrist range of motion, grip strength, and pain and DASH scores. Postoperative x-rays also were taken to assess union and screw position. At average follow-up of 98 weeks, they found that all patients returned to their preinjury level of work and 5 of 6 collegiate or professional athletes returned to unrestricted play. Pain and DASH scores demonstrated excellent functional outcomes as well. Central screw placement was achieved in all but 1 patient, and only 1 fracture failed to heal at 2 months after surgery. Other studies have found similar results and reported low complications using the volar approach,[116,117] and in comparing casting to percutaneous fixation, but with respect to fracture union, return to activity, and complications, results differ. Drac and colleagues[118] reported a lower failure rate and better range of motion and grip strength in the surgical cohort at 1 year. In contrast, Adolfsson and colleagues[119] conducted a randomized trial comparing percutaneous screw fixation with short-arm spica casting for nondisplaced scaphoid waist fractures and published differing results. Initially, the surgical group had achieved better improvements in range of motion at 4 months, but there was no difference in final motion. In addition, they found no differences in the rate or time to union or grip strength at final follow-up. In a similar study by Bond and colleagues,[120] there was no difference in functional recovery (union rate, grip strength, or motion), but surgery resulted in a faster healing times at 2-year follow-up. Bushnell and colleagues[121] evaluated complications encountered with dorsal percutaneous screw fixation in their retrospective review of 24 patients, and found a 29% overall complication rate, suggesting that surgical complications may be more common than previously thought. Moreover, Vinnars and colleagues[122] compared the results from casting and surgery at 10-year follow-up. Although they found no differences in symptoms or functional outcomes, there was a trend toward the development of scaphotrapezial arthritis in the surgical group. The differences in outcomes seen in the previously mentioned studies are largely due to heterogeneity in study design and variable patient follow-up. This makes the evidence inconclusive to recommend surgery or nonoperative management, which was also the finding in a recent meta-analysis of 6 randomized controlled trials involving 363 patients.[123]

The current evidence does not stoutly support the use of either cast immobilization or surgery for nondisplaced scaphoid fractures. A large multicenter study with long-term follow-up is needed to help determine the best method of treatment. At this time, the "optimal" management decision should be made by the surgeon and patient together after careful discussion of the patient's unique expectations, values, and goals.

EBM bottom line recommendation

The optimal management of non-displaced scaphoid fractures remains controversial.

We presented several examples of how EBM has unified clinical practice decisions and how ongoing EBM continues to shape the way in which surgeons develop patient care strategies. The underlying principle of EBM relies on robust data generated from high-quality level 1 randomized controlled studies. However, randomized controlled trials are not without shortcomings. The generation of high-quality scientific data requires the evaluation of large numbers of homogeneous patient groups. From these outcomes, generalizations are made and clinical practice guidelines emerge. But the treatment algorithms that are applied to the study target population are not necessarily appropriate for the individual patient in your office, and thus outliers may not receive optimal care. Another problem occurs in cases of rare pathology, like tumors, or in patients with congenital or posttraumatic deformities in which patient heterogeneity precludes the routine application of treatments defined from level 1 data. It is also difficult to apply the treatment recommendations from level 1 studies to atypical patient presentations of commonly encountered diseases. For example, level 1 data-derived recommendations would mandate that a 25-year-old man with history and physical examination consistent with CTS undergo CTR alone. However, in this case, it would be more prudent to perform a rheumatologic workup before surgery, particularly because this patient if diagnosed with RA may benefit from a concomitant flexor tenosynovectomy. Clinical presentations involving complex heterogeneous injury patterns (eg, a distal radius fracture with a displaced volar lunate lip fragment) represent another area in which level 4 data would be more useful in guiding patient care. Finally, in cases of systemic disease, especially where there is variability in expressivity of symptoms and anatomic sites involved, case series or case reports would better enable the physician to provide more effective patient treatment. The benefit of level 4 data under these circumstances is that careful observation and planning can provide the best evidence to design an excellent patient care plan.

In summary, using high levels of evidence is a powerful practice tool that together with one's clinical experience will enhance a surgeon's ability to select appropriate treatment and deliver quality patient care. Although level 1 studies yield the most stringent scientific results for broad application, data from case reports and case series are equally important in the management of the less prevalent, more heterogeneous clinical conditions. Even though level 1 studies provide objective data readily available at the stroke of a key or a mouse click, the study findings may not always be in alignment with one's clinical gestalt. An important principle in the practice of EBM is to consider one's own clinical expertise. This expertise evolves over years, is often not evidence based, and is not easily dismissed, even in the presence of data from quality clinical studies. So the question becomes, will doctors continue to make decisions based on anecdotal experiences or will they embrace high-level evidence studies? The answer to practicing quality EBM is a combination of the two.

REFERENCES

1. Altay T, Gunal I, Ozturk H. Local injection treatment for lateral epicondylitis. Clin Orthop Relat Res 2002;(398):127–30.
2. Lindenhovius A, Henket M, Gilligan BP, et al. Injection of dexamethasone versus placebo for lateral elbow pain: a prospective, double-blind, randomized clinical trial. J Hand Surg Am 2008; 33(6):909–19.
3. Newcomer KL, Laskowski ER, Idank DM, et al. Corticosteroid injection in early treatment of lateral epicondylitis. Clin J Sport Med 2001;11(4):214–22.
4. Smidt N, van der Windt DA, Assendelft WJ, et al. Corticosteroid injections, physiotherapy, or a wait-and-see policy for lateral epicondylitis: a randomised controlled trial. Lancet 2002;359(9307): 657–62.
5. Bisset L, Beller E, Jull G, et al. Mobilisation with movement and exercise, corticosteroid injection, or wait and see for tennis elbow: randomised trial. BMJ 2006;333(7575):939.
6. Coombes BK, Bisset L, Brooks P, et al. Effect of corticosteroid injection, physiotherapy, or both on clinical outcomes in patients with unilateral lateral epicondylalgia: a randomized controlled trial. JAMA 2013;309(5):461–9.
7. Tonks JH, Pai SK, Murali SR. Steroid injection therapy is the best conservative treatment for lateral epicondylitis: a prospective randomised controlled trial. Int J Clin Pract 2007;61(2):240–6.
8. Barr S, Cerisola FL, Blanchard V. Effectiveness of corticosteroid injections compared with physiotherapeutic interventions for lateral epicondylitis: a systematic review. Physiotherapy 2009;95(4): 251–65.
9. Coombes BK, Bisset L, Vicenzino B. Efficacy and safety of corticosteroid injections and other injections for management of tendinopathy: a systematic review of randomised controlled trials. Lancet 2010;376(9754):1751–67.
10. Krogh TP, Bartels EM, Ellingsen T, et al. Comparative effectiveness of injection therapies in lateral epicondylitis: a systematic review and network meta-analysis of randomized controlled trials. Am J Sports Med 2013;41(6):1435–46.
11. Stefanou A, Marshall N, Holdan W, et al. A randomized study comparing corticosteroid injection to corticosteroid iontophoresis for lateral epicondylitis. J Hand Surg Am 2012;37(1):104–9.
12. Nichols AW. Complications associated with the use of corticosteroids in the treatment of athletic injuries. Clin J Sport Med 2005;15(5):370–5.
13. Nirschl RP, Pettrone FA. Tennis elbow. The surgical treatment of lateral epicondylitis. J Bone Joint Surg Am 1979;61(6A):832–9.
14. Scott A, Khan KM. Corticosteroids: short-term gain for long-term pain? Lancet 2010;376(9754): 1714–5.
15. Lin YC, Tu YK, Chen SS, et al. Comparison between botulinum toxin and corticosteroid injection in the treatment of acute and subacute tennis elbow: a prospective, randomized, double-blind, active drug-controlled pilot study. Am J Phys Med Rehabil 2010;89(8):653–9.
16. Bellapianta J, Swartz F, Lisella J, et al. Randomized prospective evaluation of injection techniques for the treatment of lateral epicondylitis. Orthopedics 2011;34(11):e708–12.
17. Krogh TP, Fredberg U, Stengaard-Pedersen K, et al. Treatment of lateral epicondylitis with platelet-rich plasma, glucocorticoid, or saline: a randomized, double-blind, placebo-controlled trial. Am J Sports Med 2013;41(3):625–35.
18. Gosens T, Peerbooms JC, van Laar W, et al. Ongoing positive effect of platelet-rich plasma versus corticosteroid injection in lateral epicondylitis: a double-blind randomized controlled trial with 2-year follow-up. Am J Sports Med 2011;39(6): 1200–8.
19. Peerbooms JC, Sluimer J, Bruijn DJ, et al. Positive effect of an autologous platelet concentrate in lateral epicondylitis in a double-blind randomized controlled trial: platelet-rich plasma versus corticosteroid injection with a 1-year follow-up. Am J Sports Med 2010;38(2):255–62.
20. Carayannopoulos A, Borg-Stein J, Sokolof J, et al. Prolotherapy versus corticosteroid injections for the treatment of lateral epicondylosis: a randomized controlled trial. PM R 2011;3(8): 706–15.
21. Kazemi M, Azma K, Tavana B, et al. Autologous blood versus corticosteroid local injection in the short-term treatment of lateral elbow tendinopathy: a randomized clinical trial of efficacy. Am J Phys Med Rehabil 2010;89(8):660–7.
22. Wolf JM, Ozer K, Scott F, et al. Comparison of autologous blood, corticosteroid, and saline injection in the treatment of lateral epicondylitis: a prospective, randomized, controlled multicenter study. J Hand Surg Am 2011;36(8):1269–72.

23. Trinh KV, Phillips SD, Ho E, et al. Acupuncture for the alleviation of lateral epicondyle pain: a systematic review. Rheumatology (Oxford) 2004;43(9): 1085–90.

24. Gunduz R, Malas FÜ, Borman P, et al. Physical therapy, corticosteroid injection, and extracorporeal shock wave treatment in lateral epicondylitis. Clinical and ultrasonographical comparison. Clin Rheumatol 2012;31(5):807–12.

25. Hanssen AD, Amadio PC, DeSilva SP, et al. Deep postoperative wound infection after carpal tunnel release. J Hand Surg Am 1989;14(5):869–73.

26. Harness NG, Inacio MC, Pfeil FF, et al. Rate of infection after carpal tunnel release surgery and effect of antibiotic prophylaxis. J Hand Surg Am 2010;35(2):189–96.

27. Kleinert JM, Hoffmann J, Miller Crain G, et al. Postoperative infection in a double-occupancy operating room. A prospective study of two thousand four hundred and fifty-eight procedures on the extremities. J Bone Joint Surg Am 1997;79(4): 503–13.

28. Tosti R, Fowler J, Dwyer J, et al. Is antibiotic prophylaxis necessary in elective soft tissue hand surgery? Orthopedics 2012;35(6):e829–33.

29. Aydin N, Uraloğlu M, Yılmaz Burhanoğlu AD, et al. A prospective trial on the use of antibiotics in hand surgery. Plast Reconstr Surg 2010;126(5):1617–23.

30. Bykowski MR, Sivak WN, Cray J, et al. Assessing the impact of antibiotic prophylaxis in outpatient elective hand surgery: a single-center, retrospective review of 8,850 cases. J Hand Surg Am 2011;36(11):1741–7.

31. Savage R. In vitro studies of a new method of flexor tendon repair. J Hand Surg Br 1985;10(2):135–41.

32. Urbaniak JR, Cahill JD, Mortenson RA. Tendon suture methods: analysis of tensile strength, in AAOS Symposium on Tendon Surgery in the Hand. St Louis (MO): Mosby; 1975. p. 70–80.

33. Alavanja G, Dailey E, Mass DP. Repair of zone II flexor digitorum profundus lacerations using varying suture sizes: a comparative biomechanical study. J Hand Surg Am 2005;30(3):448–54.

34. McLarney E, Hoffman H, Wolfe SW. Biomechanical analysis of the cruciate four-strand flexor tendon repair. J Hand Surg Am 1999;24(2):295–301.

35. Savage R, Risitano G. Flexor tendon repair using a "six strand" method of repair and early active mobilisation. J Hand Surg Br 1989;14(4):396–9.

36. Su BW, Raia FJ, Quitkin HM, et al. Gross and histological analysis of healing after dog flexor tendon repair with the Teno Fix device. J Hand Surg Br 2006;31(5):524–9.

37. Tang JB, Gu YT, Rice K, et al. Evaluation of four methods of flexor tendon repair for postoperative active mobilization. Plast Reconstr Surg 2001; 107(3):742–9.

38. Thurman RT, Trumble TE, Hanel DP, et al. Two-, four-, and six-strand zone II flexor tendon repairs: an in situ biomechanical comparison using a cadaver model. J Hand Surg Am 1998;23(2): 261–5.

39. Tang JB, Wang B, Chen F, et al. Biomechanical evaluation of flexor tendon repair techniques. Clin Orthop Relat Res 2001;(386):252–9.

40. Stein T, Ali A, Hamman J, et al. A randomized biomechanical study of zone II human flexor tendon repairs analyzed in an in vitro model. J Hand Surg Am 1998;23(6):1046–51.

41. Wade PJ, Wetherell RG, Amis AA. Flexor tendon repair: significant gain in strength from the Halsted peripheral suture technique. J Hand Surg Br 1989; 14(2):232–5.

42. Hatanaka H, Manske PR. Effect of the cross-sectional area of locking loops in flexor tendon repair. J Hand Surg Am 1999;24(4):751–60.

43. Hatanaka H, Zhang J, Manske PR. An in vivo study of locking and grasping techniques using a passive mobilization protocol in experimental animals. J Hand Surg Am 2000;25(2):260–9.

44. Hoffmann GL, Buchler U, Vogelin E. Clinical results of flexor tendon repair in zone II using a six-strand double-loop technique compared with a two-strand technique. J Hand Surg Eur Vol 2008; 33(4):418–23.

45. Osada D, Fujita S, Tamai K, et al. Flexor tendon repair in zone II with 6-strand techniques and early active mobilization. J Hand Surg Am 2006;31(6): 987–92.

46. Mashadi ZB, Amis AA. Variation of holding strength of synthetic absorbable flexor tendon sutures with time. J Hand Surg Br 1992;17(3):278–81.

47. Caulfield RH, Maleki-Tabrizi A, Patel H, et al. Comparison of zones 1 to 4 flexor tendon repairs using absorbable and unabsorbable four-strand core sutures. J Hand Surg Eur Vol 2008;33(4):412–7.

48. Su BW, Solomons M, Barrow A, et al. Device for zone-II flexor tendon repair. A multicenter, randomized, blinded, clinical trial. J Bone Joint Surg Am 2005;87(5):923–35.

49. Rocchi L, Merolli A, Genzini A, et al. Flexor tendon injuries of the hand treated with TenoFix: mid-term results. J Orthop Traumatol 2008;9(4):201–8.

50. Su BW, Protopsaltis TS, Koff MF, et al. The biomechanical analysis of a tendon fixation device for flexor tendon repair. J Hand Surg Am 2005;30(2): 237–45.

51. Wolfe SW, Willis AA, Campbell D, et al. Biomechanic comparison of the Teno Fix tendon repair device with the cruciate and modified Kessler techniques. J Hand Surg Am 2007;32(3):356–66.

52. Bhatia R, Field J, Grote J, et al. Does splintage help pain after carpal tunnel release? J Hand Surg Br 2000;25(2):150.

53. Bury TF, Akelman E, Weiss AP. Prospective, randomized trial of splinting after carpal tunnel release. Ann Plast Surg 1995;35(1):19–22.

54. Finsen V, Andersen K, Russwurm H. No advantage from splinting the wrist after open carpal tunnel release. A randomized study of 82 wrists. Acta Orthop Scand 1999;70(3):288–92.

55. Huemer GM, Koller M, Pachinger T, et al. Postoperative splinting after open carpal tunnel release does not improve functional and neurological outcome. Muscle Nerve 2007;36(4):528–31.

56. Cook AC, Szabo RM, Birkholz SW, et al. Early mobilization following carpal tunnel release. A prospective randomized study. J Hand Surg Br 1995; 20(2):228–30.

57. Henry SL, Hubbard BA, Concannon MJ. Splinting after carpal tunnel release: current practice, scientific evidence, and trends. Plast Reconstr Surg 2008; 122(4):1095–9.

58. Duncan KH, Lewis RC Jr, Foreman KA, et al. Treatment of carpal tunnel syndrome by members of the American Society for Surgery of the Hand: results of a questionnaire. J Hand Surg Am 1987; 12(3):384–91.

59. Levis CM, Tung TH, Mackinnon SE. Variations in incisions and postoperative management in carpal tunnel surgery. Can J Plast Surg 2002;10(63):63–7.

60. Keith MW, Masear V, Chung KC, et al. American Academy of Orthopaedic Surgeons Clinical Practice Guideline on diagnosis of carpal tunnel syndrome. J Bone Joint Surg Am 2009;91(10):2478–9.

61. Gervasio O, Gambardella G, Zaccone C, et al. Simple decompression versus anterior submuscular transposition of the ulnar nerve in severe cubital tunnel syndrome: a prospective randomized study. Neurosurgery 2005;56(1):108–17 [discussion: 117].

62. Biggs M, Curtis JA. Randomized, prospective study comparing ulnar neurolysis in situ with submuscular transposition. Neurosurgery 2006;58(2): 296–304 [discussion: 296–304].

63. Bartels RH, Verhagen WI, van der Wilt GJ, et al. Prospective randomized controlled study comparing simple decompression versus anterior subcutaneous transposition for idiopathic neuropathy of the ulnar nerve at the elbow: part 1. Neurosurgery 2005;56(3):522–30 [discussion: 522–30].

64. Macadam SA, Gandhi R, Bezuhly M, et al. Simple decompression versus anterior subcutaneous and submuscular transposition of the ulnar nerve for cubital tunnel syndrome: a meta-analysis. J Hand Surg Am 2008;33(8):1314.e1–12.

65. Zlowodzki M, Chan S, Bhandari M, et al. Anterior transposition compared with simple decompression for treatment of cubital tunnel syndrome. A meta-analysis of randomized, controlled trials. J Bone Joint Surg Am 2007;89(12):2591–8.

66. Martou G, Veltri K, Thoma A. Surgical treatment of osteoarthritis of the carpometacarpal joint of the thumb: a systematic review. Plast Reconstr Surg 2004;114(2):421–32.

67. Wajon A, Ada L, Edmunds I. Surgery for thumb (trapeziometacarpal joint) osteoarthritis. Cochrane Database Syst Rev 2005;(4):CD004631.

68. Wajon A, Carr E, Edmunds I, et al. Surgery for thumb (trapeziometacarpal joint) osteoarthritis. Cochrane Database Syst Rev 2009;(4):CD004631.

69. Vermeulen GM, Slijper H, Feitz R, et al. Surgical management of primary thumb carpometacarpal osteoarthritis: a systematic review. J Hand Surg Am 2011;36(1):157–69.

70. Davis TR, Pace A. Trapeziectomy for trapeziometacarpal joint osteoarthritis: is ligament reconstruction and temporary stabilisation of the pseudarthrosis with a Kirschner wire important? J Hand Surg Eur Vol 2009;34(3):312–21.

71. Gray KV, Meals RA. Hematoma and distraction arthroplasty for thumb basal joint osteoarthritis: minimum 6.5-year follow-up evaluation. J Hand Surg Am 2007;32(1):23–9.

72. Wolf JM, Delaronde S. Current trends in nonoperative and operative treatment of trapeziometacarpal osteoarthritis: a survey of US hand surgeons. J Hand Surg Am 2012;37(1):77–82.

73. Hershman SH, Immerman I, Bechtel C, et al. The effects of pronator quadratus repair on outcomes after volar plating of distal radius fractures. J Orthop Trauma 2013;27(3):130–3.

74. Ahsan ZS, Yao J. The importance of pronator quadratus repair in the treatment of distal radius fractures with volar plating. Hand (N Y) 2012;7(3): 276–80.

75. Swigart CR, Badon MA, Bruegel VL, et al. Assessment of pronator quadratus repair integrity following volar plate fixation for distal radius fractures: a prospective clinical cohort study. J Hand Surg Am 2012;37(9):1868–73.

76. Tosti R, Ilyas AM. Prospective evaluation of pronator quadratus repair following volar plate fixation of distal radius fractures. J Hand Surg Am 2013; 38(9):1678–84.

77. Scholten RJ, Mink van der Molen A, Uitdehaag BM, et al. Surgical treatment options for carpal tunnel syndrome. Cochrane Database Syst Rev 2007;(4):CD003905.

78. Atroshi I, Larsson GU, Ornstein E, et al. Outcomes of endoscopic surgery compared with open surgery for carpal tunnel syndrome among employed patients: randomised controlled trial. BMJ 2006; 332(7556):1473.

79. Jacobsen MB, Rahme H. A prospective, randomized study with an independent observer comparing open carpal tunnel release with endoscopic carpal tunnel release. J Hand Surg Br 1996;21(2):202–4.

80. Saw NL, Jones S, Shepstone L, et al. Early outcome and cost-effectiveness of endoscopic versus open carpal tunnel release: a randomized prospective trial. J Hand Surg Br 2003; 28(5):444–9.

81. Kieth MW, Masear V, Amadio P, et al. Treatment of carpal tunnel syndrome. J Am Acad Orthop Surgeons 2009;17(6):397–405.

82. Atroshi I, Hofer M, Larsson GU, et al. Open compared with 2-portal endoscopic carpal tunnel release: a 5-year follow-up of a randomized controlled trial. J Hand Surg Am 2009;34(2): 266–72.

83. Dammers JW, Veering MM, Vermeulen M. Injection with methylprednisolone proximal to the carpal tunnel: randomised double blind trial. BMJ 1999; 319(7214):884–6.

84. Armstrong T, Devor W, Borschel L, et al. Intracarpal steroid injection is safe and effective for short-term management of carpal tunnel syndrome. Muscle Nerve 2004;29(1):82–8.

85. Visser LH, Ngo Q, Groeneweg SJ, et al. Long term effect of local corticosteroid injection for carpal tunnel syndrome: a relation with electrodiagnostic severity. Clin Neurophysiol 2012;123(4): 838–41.

86. Wong SM, Hui AC, Lo SK, et al. Single vs. two steroid injections for carpal tunnel syndrome: a randomised clinical trial. Int J Clin Pract 2005; 59(12):1417–21.

87. Sevim S, Dogu O, Camdeviren H, et al. Long-term effectiveness of steroid injections and splinting in mild and moderate carpal tunnel syndrome. Neurol Sci 2004;25(2):48–52.

88. Habib GS, Badarny S, Rawashdeh H. A novel approach of local corticosteroid injection for the treatment of carpal tunnel syndrome. Clin Rheumatol 2006;25(3):338–40.

89. O'Gradaigh D, Merry P. Corticosteroid injection for the treatment of carpal tunnel syndrome. Ann Rheum Dis 2000;59(11):918–9.

90. Catalano LW 3rd, Glickel SZ, Barron OA, et al. Effect of local corticosteroid injection of the hand and wrist on blood glucose in patients with diabetes mellitus. Orthopedics 2012;35(12):e1754–8.

91. Vahi PS, Kals M, Kõiv L, et al. Preoperative corticosteroid injections are associated with worse long-term outcome of surgical carpal tunnel release. Acta Orthop 2014;85(1):102–6.

92. de Mos M, van der Windt AE, Jahr H, et al. Can platelet-rich plasma enhance tendon repair? A cell culture study. Am J Sports Med 2008;36(6): 1171–8.

93. Morizaki Y, Zhao C, An KN, et al. The effects of platelet-rich plasma on bone marrow stromal cell transplants for tendon healing in vitro. J Hand Surg Am 2010;35(11):1833–41.

94. Bosch G, Moleman M, Barneveld A, et al. The effect of platelet-rich plasma on the neovascularization of surgically created equine superficial digital flexor tendon lesions. Scand J Med Sci Sports 2011;21(4):554–61.

95. Sato D, Takahara M, Narita A, et al. Effect of platelet-rich plasma with fibrin matrix on healing of intrasynovial flexor tendons. J Hand Surg Am 2012;37(7):1356–63.

96. Waljee JF, Chung KC. Objective functional outcomes and patient satisfaction after silicone metacarpophalangeal arthroplasty for rheumatoid arthritis. J Hand Surg Am 2012;37(1):47–54.

97. Chung KC, Burke FD, Wilgis EF, et al. A prospective study comparing outcomes after reconstruction in rheumatoid arthritis patients with severe ulnar drift deformities. Plast Reconstr Surg 2009;123(6):1769–77.

98. Chung KC, Kowalski CP, Myra Kim H, et al. Patient outcomes following Swanson silastic metacarpophalangeal joint arthroplasty in the rheumatoid hand: a systematic overview. J Rheumatol 2000;27(6):1395–402.

99. Chung KC, Kotsis SV, Kim HM. A prospective outcomes study of Swanson metacarpophalangeal joint arthroplasty for the rheumatoid hand. J Hand Surg Am 2004;29(4):646–53.

100. Schmidt K, Willburger RE, Miehlke RK, et al. Ten-year follow-up of silicone arthroplasty of the metacarpophalangeal joints in rheumatoid hands. Scand J Plast Reconstr Surg Hand Surg 1999; 33(4):433–8.

101. Kirschenbaum D, Schneider LH, Adams DC, et al. Arthroplasty of the metacarpophalangeal joints with use of silicone-rubber implants in patients who have rheumatoid arthritis. Long-term results. J Bone Joint Surg Am 1993;75(1):3–12.

102. Olsen I, Gebuhr P, Sonne-Holm S. Silastic arthroplasty in rheumatoid MCP-joints. 60 joints followed for 7 years. Acta Orthop Scand 1994;65(4):430–1.

103. Wilson YG, Sykes PJ, Niranjan NS. Long-term follow-up of Swanson's silastic arthroplasty of the metacarpophalangeal joints in rheumatoid arthritis. J Hand Surg Br 1993;18(1):81–91.

104. Goldfarb CA, Stern PJ. Metacarpophalangeal joint arthroplasty in rheumatoid arthritis. A long-term assessment. J Bone Joint Surg Am 2003;85(10): 1869–78.

105. Handoll HH, Huntley JS, Madhok R. Different methods of external fixation for treating distal radial fractures in adults. Cochrane Database Syst Rev 2008;(1):CD006522.

106. Handoll HH, Vaghela MV, Madhok R. Percutaneous pinning for treating distal radial fractures in adults. Cochrane Database Syst Rev 2007;(3):CD006080.

107. Handoll HH, Madhok R. From evidence to best practice in the management of fractures of the

distal radius in adults: working towards a research agenda. BMC Musculoskelet Disord 2003;4:27.

108. Wright TW, Horodyski M, Smith DW. Functional outcome of unstable distal radius fractures: ORIF with a volar fixed-angle tine plate versus external fixation. J Hand Surg Am 2005;30(2):289–99.

109. Jeudy J, Steiger V, Boyer P, et al. Treatment of complex fractures of the distal radius: a prospective randomised comparison of external fixation 'versus' locked volar plating. Injury 2012;43(2): 174–9.

110. Walenkamp MM, Bentohami A, Beerekamp MS, et al. Functional outcome in patients with unstable distal radius fractures, volar locking plate versus external fixation: a meta-analysis. Strategies Trauma Limb Reconstr 2013;8(2):67–75.

111. Esposito J, Schemitsch EH, Saccone M, et al. External fixation versus open reduction with plate fixation for distal radius fractures: a meta-analysis of randomised controlled trials. Injury 2013;44(4): 409–16.

112. Wei DH, Poolman RW, Bhandari M, et al. External fixation versus internal fixation for unstable distal radius fractures: a systematic review and meta-analysis of comparative clinical trials. J Orthop Trauma 2012;26(7):386–94.

113. Wang J, Yang Y, Ma J, et al. Open reduction and internal fixation versus external fixation for unstable distal radial fractures: a meta-analysis. Orthop Traumatol Surg Res 2013;99(3):321–31.

114. Grewal R, MacDermid JC, King GJ, et al. Open reduction internal fixation versus percutaneous pinning with external fixation of distal radius fractures: a prospective, randomized clinical trial. J Hand Surg Am 2011;36(12):1899–906.

115. Bedi A, Jebson PJ, Hayden RJ, et al. Internal fixation of acute, nondisplaced scaphoid waist fractures via a limited dorsal approach: an assessment of radiographic and functional outcomes. J Hand Surg Am 2007;32(3):326–33.

116. Wozasek GE, Moser KD. Percutaneous screw fixation for fractures of the scaphoid. J Bone Joint Surg Br 1991;73(1):138–42.

117. Ledoux P, Chahidi N, Moermans JP, et al. Percutaneous Herbert screw osteosynthesis of the scaphoid bone. Acta Orthop Belg 1995;61(1): 43–7 [in French].

118. Drac P, Manak P, Labonek I. Percutaneous osteosynthesis versus cast immobilisation for the treatment of minimally and non-displaced scaphoid fractures. Functional outcomes after a follow-up of at least 12 months. Biomed Pap Med Fac Univ Palacky Olomouc Czech Repub 2005; 149(1):149–51.

119. Adolfsson L, Lindau T, Arner M. Acutrak screw fixation versus cast immobilisation for undisplaced scaphoid waist fractures. J Hand Surg Br 2001; 26(3):192–5.

120. Bond CD, Shin AY, McBride MT, et al. Percutaneous screw fixation or cast immobilization for nondisplaced scaphoid fractures. J Bone Joint Surg Am 2001;83(4):483–8.

121. Bushnell BD, McWilliams AD, Messer TM. Complications in dorsal percutaneous cannulated screw fixation of nondisplaced scaphoid waist fractures. J Hand Surg Am 2007;32(6):827–33.

122. Vinnars B, Pietreanu M, Bodestedt A, et al. Nonoperative compared with operative treatment of acute scaphoid fractures. A randomized clinical trial. J Bone Joint Surgery Am 2008;90(6):1176–85.

123. Ibrahim T, Qureshi A, Sutton AJ, et al. Surgical versus nonsurgical treatment of acute minimally displaced and undisplaced scaphoid waist fractures: pairwise and network meta-analyses of randomized controlled trials. J Hand Surg Am 2011; 36(11):1759–68.e1.

Measuring and Understanding Treatment Effectiveness in Hand Surgery

Sophocles H. Voineskos, MD, MSc[a,b,*],
Christopher J. Coroneos, MD[a,b],
Achilleas Thoma, MD, MSc, FRCSC[a,b,c],
Mohit Bhandari, MD, PhD, FRCSC[c,d]

KEYWORDS

- Hand surgery • Treatment outcome • Comparative effectiveness research • Relative risk • *P*-value
- Confidence interval • Minimal clinically important difference • Number needed to treat

KEY POINTS

- The randomized controlled trial is the reference standard study design when comparing 2 therapeutic interventions.
- Before interpreting study results, the methodology of the trial must be assessed to ensure there were no errors in design or execution that might invalidate the results.
- Absolute and relative measures of treatment effectiveness assist in the interpretation of study results.
- Valid and reliable patient-important outcome measures in hand surgery exist and should be used to assess outcomes.
- Study findings should be interpreted within the clinical context, and preference, of the individual patient being treated.

INTRODUCTION

In 1992, evidence-based medicine (EBM) was introduced as a shift in medical paradigms.[1] The demand for a rational decision-making process in health care has increased the importance of using EBM to enhance the traditional skills of clinical practice. Today, rational application of EBM principles to hand surgery research is not only recommended, but expected if surgeons are to identify and appraise best evidence.[2]

Evidence-based hand surgery posits that clinicians should be using the best evidence available when managing their patients, even if the quality of that evidence is limited.[3] In-depth background knowledge and sound clinical decision making are more important than ever, as evidence of

Conflicts of Interest: The authors state that they have no conflicts of interest or financial disclosures. No funds were received for the preparation of this article.

[a] Division of Plastic and Reconstructive Surgery, Department of Surgery, McMaster University, HSC 4E12, 1200 Main Street West, Hamilton, Ontario L8N 3Z5, Canada; [b] Surgical Outcomes Research Centre (SOURCE), McMaster University, 202-39 Charlton Avenue East, Hamilton, Ontario L8N 1Y3, Canada; [c] Department of Clinical Epidemiology and Biostatistics, McMaster University HSC 2C, 1280 Main Street West, Hamilton, Ontario L8S 4K1, Canada; [d] Division of Orthopaedic Surgery, Department of Surgery, McMaster University, Well-Health Building, 293 Wellington Street North, Hamilton, Ontario L8L 8E7, Canada

* Corresponding author. Division of Plastic and Reconstructive Surgery, Department of Surgery, McMaster University, HSC 4E12, 1200 Main Street West, Hamilton, Ontario L8N 3Z5.

E-mail address: sophocles.voineskos@medportal.ca

http://dx.doi.org/10.1016/j.hcl.2014.04.008
0749-0712/14/$ – see front matter © 2014 Elsevier Inc. All rights reserved.

hand.theclinics.com

treatment effectiveness does not automatically imply that the treatment should be administered.

Applying EBM principles for an intervention aids surgeons in choosing the most appropriate surgical procedure for a particular patient. Surgeons need the tools to assess the strength and usefulness of the available evidence and to evaluate the measurement and treatment effectiveness of an outcome. This process will allow us to defend therapeutic interventions based on available evidence and not anecdote.[4]

In a randomized controlled trial (RCT), individuals are randomly allocated to treatment groups and followed to determine the effect of the therapeutic intervention on one or more outcomes. The advantage of a methodologically sound RCT is the ability to balance both known and unknown prognostic factors between the 2 comparison groups.[3]

Conversely, in a nonrandomized (observational) study, the deliberate choice of treatment of each patient implies that the observed outcome may be a result of differences among the patients undergoing treatment, rather than the treatment itself.[4] The potential roles of observational studies in hand surgery have been discussed previously.[5] With an appropriate research question, and recognition of inherent limitations, the observational study can be used effectively in hand surgery.[5]

This article uses a practical example to demonstrate how evidence-based surgery concepts are used to interpret and apply the results of an RCT in hand surgery.

CLINICAL SCENARIO

Mr W. White is a 57-year-old man with Dupuytren disease. On examination, he has a metacarpophalangeal joint contracture of 35° of his ring finger and an easily palpable palmar cord over the ring metacarpal. The patient states that a family member, who is in the medical field, provided him with a relevant publication to pass along to you and recommended he request a limited fasciectomy (LF) treatment of his Dupuytren contracture. He produces a printed copy of the following RCT by van Rijssen and colleagues[6]: "Five-year results of a randomized clinical trial on treatment in Dupuytren disease percutaneous needle fasciotomy versus limited fasciectomy."

The publication provided to you describes an RCT including 111 patients, with 115 affected hands, with a minimal passive extension deficit of 30° and the existence of a clearly defined palmar cord. Participants were randomly allocated to percutaneous needle fasciotomy (PNF) or LF. The primary outcome was disease recurrence.[6]

ASSESSING THE METHODOLOGY OF THE TRIAL

This article focuses on interpreting treatment effectiveness and applying the results of the trial to your patient. However, before using results from an RCT, the methodology of the trial must be assessed to ensure the trial's validity. The methodological assessment of this RCT has been summarized in **Box 1**. The detailed guide to answer the question "Are the results valid?" for a study comparing therapeutic interventions can be found in "Users' Guides to the Medical Literature"[3] and in the "Users' Guide to the Surgical Literature".[7] Furthermore, a discussion on specific challenges for RCT methodology in hand surgery is available.[8]

IMPORTANT CONCEPTS IN INTERPRETING TREATMENT EFFECTIVENESS
How Large was the Treatment Effect?

The primary outcome in van Rijssen and associates' RCT[6] is recurrence of disease. This outcome is dichotomous, in which the patient either has an event or he does not.[6]

In the van Rijssen and associates' RCT,[6] 23.3% of the LF group developed recurrence (with one of these patients developing extension of disease). In the PNF group, 84.9% of patients developed recurrence.[6] These results can be expressed as a risk difference, relative risk (RR), or relative risk reduction (RRR) (**Box 2**).

The absolute difference is also known as *absolute risk reduction* (ARR) or risk difference. The ARR is the difference between the proportion who had recurrence in the LF group (0.233) and the proportion who had recurrence in the PNF group (0.849), or PNF − LF = 0.849 − 0.233 = 0.616, or 62%. This measure of effect uses absolute, rather than relative, terms to compare the proportion of patients who experienced recurrence.

When weighing benefit and harm, concept of a *number needed to treat* (NNT) is used. The NNT is the number of patients a surgeon must treat to create one positive outcome (see section *Are the Likely Treatment Benefits worth the Potential Harm?* for further discussion of NNT).

Another way to express the impact of the treatment is through an RR. The RR represents the risk of recurrence among patients who received LF relative to those who received PNF, or LF/PNF = 0.233/0.849 = 0.274, or 27%. To interpret this RR, the risk of recurrence when undergoing LF is about one-quarter that of PNF.

When using a dichotomous outcome, the most commonly reported measure of a treatment effect is the complement of the *RR*, which is the RRR. It

Box 1
Key features of the RCT: LF versus PNF

Question	Answer	Details
Did intervention and control groups start with the same prognosis?		
Were patients randomized?	Yes	Performed by drawing of lots
Was randomization concealed?	Partially	Assignment envelopes were numbered, but no mention of being sealed or opaque
Were patients in the study groups similar with respect to known prognostic factors?	Yes	Baseline characteristics displayed for reader
Was prognostic balance maintained as the study progressed?		
Were patients blinded?	Probably not	Not mentioned. PNF occurred in "outpatient treatment room". LF occurred in "surgical theater"
Were outcome assessors blinded?	No	Measurements taken by the surgeon
Were surgeons blinded?	No	Not possible
Did the investigators take into consideration the learning curve?	Unknown	Information is not included in the manuscript
Were the groups prognostically balanced at the study's completion?		
Was follow-up complete?	No, but had 5 year outcome	121 patients were randomized, 93 patients were included in the final analysis. This trial had a follow-up rate of 76.8% for a 5 year outcome
Were patients analyzed in the groups to which they were randomized?	Yes	
Was the trial stopped early?	No	

Data from van Rijssen AL, ter Linden H, Werker PM. Five-year results of a randomized clinical trial on treatment in Dupuytren's disease: percutaneous needle fasciotomy versus limited fasciectomy. Plast Reconstr Surg 2012;129(2):467–77.

is expressed as a percent: RRR = (1 − LF/PNF) × 100% = (1 − 0.274) × 100% = 76.2%, or 76%. An RRR of 76% means that LF reduced the risk of revision surgery by 76% relative to that occurring among patients who underwent PNF. The greater the RRR, the more effective is the intervention.

The results section of the van Rijssen and associates' RCT[6] also displays the RR of recurrence over time in a *survival analysis* (the Kaplan-Meier survival estimate). The weighted RR over the entire study is called a *hazard ratio*, which represents the instantaneous risk over the study time period.

The discussed relative measures of treatment effect (RR and RRR) are commonly used. However, it is important to differentiate between the absolute measure (ARR), and the relative measures (RR, RRR). Although not the case in the van Rijssen and associates' RCT,[6] there are occasions when simply stating an RRR can be deceptive.

For example, if the recurrence rate of Dupuytren disease when performing a PNF is 50% and when performing an LF is 25%, then the *RRR* is calculated to be 50%, which is impressive.

However, if the recurrence rate of Dupuytren disease was rare, for example 2% in the PNF group and 1% in the LF group, the *RRR* is also 50%. In this example, simply interpreting the results with a relative measure of treatment effect is misleading. The corresponding ARR of recurrence of disease of 1% is no longer as exciting or likely to change your clinical practice.

How Precise was the Estimate of Treatment Effect?

The true risk reduction of a treatment of a population is unknown. The risk reduction of Dupuytren recurrence (see **Box 2**) provided by the

Box 2
Understanding treatment effectiveness in the van Rijssen and associates' RCT

Exposure	Outcome at 5 Years		
	Recurrence	No Recurrence	Total
LF	10[a]	33	43
PNF	8	45	53

PNF risk: 8/53 = 84.9%.
LF risk: 10/43 = 23.3%.
Absolute risk reduction or risk difference (ARR) = PNF − LF = 84.9% − 23.3% = 61.6%, or 62%.
Relative risk (RR) = LF/PNF = (10/43)/(8/53) × 100% = 27.4% or 27%.
Relative risk reduction (RRR) = [1 − (LF/PNF)] × 100% = 1 − 27.4% = 72.6% or 73%.
Number Needed to Treat (NNT) = 1/ARR = 1/0.616 = 1.6, or 2.
[a] In the LF group, one of the 10 patients with recurrence had extension of the disease.

Data from van Rijssen AL, ter Linden H, Werker PM. Five-year results of a randomized clinical trial on treatment in Dupuytren's disease: percutaneous needle fasciotomy versus limited fasciectomy. Plast Reconstr Surg 2012;129(2):467–77.

results of the van Rijssen and associates' RCT[6] is a *point estimate* based on data from a sample of patients recruited from the general population.

The *P-value* is often used by investigators to determine statistical significance, with a conventional threshold of 0.05. A *P-value* of .05 represents a probability of 1 in 20 that the observed effect is due to chance alone, when there is no relationship between the treatment and outcome.

The van Rijssen and associates' RCT[6] reports a difference in recurrence rate between the 2 surgical interventions of *P*<.001. This result is interpreted as a statistically significant difference between the 2 groups; the recurrence rate of Dupuytren disease after 5 years in the PNF group is significantly higher than in the LF group.

Unfortunately, there are limitations to the concept of a *P-value*. Dichotomy is introduced in the form of labeling a study as "positive" or "negative" when a *P-value* is used.[3] The drawback of the "yes/no" dichotomy is obvious when considering a trial outcome with a *P-value* of .049. This trial would be considered a "positive" trial, but how different is this result from 0.05? or a "negative" trial that might not receive as much attention with a *P-value* of .051? In many cases, the difference in these examples can be attributed to a single event, demonstrating the potential fragility of the analysis this *P-value* represents. Furthermore, the

P-value is unable to measure the strength of an association.[2]

A *confidence interval* (CI) provides the range of values within which, given the trial data, the true effect might actually lie.[9] The CI defines the range that includes the true risk reduction for a given probability, assuming the RCT was methodologically sound.

Conventionally, a 95% CI is used and can be interpreted as the range of values the investigators believe, with 95% certainty, that the true population value lies.[9] Therefore, this also means they believe there is a 5% chance that the calculated CI did not encompass the true treatment effect.

Unfortunately, the CI is not provided around the treatment effect in the van Rijssen and associates' RCT.[6] Although a CI of "1.597 to 2.628" is referenced by the investigators after reporting the *P-value*, it is not clear to the reader what this CI represents.

In general, as sample size increases in a trial, the number of outcome events increases, and there is a greater likelihood that the treatment effect observed in the trial converges with the true treatment effect.[3] Therefore, more precision (narrower CIs) can result from larger sample sizes.

CIs can help avoid the dichotomy of considering a trial "positive" or "negative". A CI can demonstrate the magnitude and direction of a treatment effect and help to determine clinical significance.

In a "positive" trial, the CI can tell you if the sample size was adequate and results are definitive, or nondefinitive and further trials are required. Likewise, in a "negative" trial, the CI can be used to determine whether the sample size was adequate and the trial results definitely negative, or nondefinitive and further trials are required.[3]

Are the Results Clinically Significant?

A trial can demonstrate a statistically significant difference between treatment groups, yet this difference may not be of clinical significance to the patient. Owing to the precision gained from extremely large sample sizes, a statistically significant result may in fact represent a clinically trivial change in the patient's outcome. Again using the hypothetical example mentioned earlier where the recurrence rates for PNF and LF were rare and differed by only 1%, if the study was conducted in many thousands of patients and yielded statistically significant results, it indicates lower recurrence in the LF group. Would you change your clinical practice and abandon PNF entirely because of the "significant" difference in recurrence rates?

Judgment of the appropriateness of the primary outcome chosen is also required. The dichotomous primary outcome, recurrence of Dupuytren disease, is a patient-important outcome. As discussed earlier, the change in *ARR* for a dichotomous outcome should be substantial. A large change in *ARR*, 62%, (see **Box 2**) is demonstrated in the van Rijssen and associates' RCT.[6] The result of the primary outcome is therefore clinically significant.

A continuous primary outcome can provide rich information. The *minimal clinically important difference* (MCID) is a measure of a clinically important, or relevant, change in health[10] in a continuous outcome. The MCID is the smallest difference in outcome score that patients perceive as beneficial enough that would mandate, in the absence of side effects or excessive cost, a change in the patient's health care management.[3,9,10]

Effect size is a measure of the strength of the relationship between the intervention and the outcome.[11] It is calculated by taking the difference in mean scores between the 2 intervention groups and dividing by the standard deviation (SD) of the scores in the control group (or the pooled SD of the treatment and control groups) (Effect Size = $(\mu_{treatment} - \mu_{control})/SD$).[3] Cohen provided a general rule of thumb when interpreting the magnitude of an effect size, approximately 0.2 being a small change, approximately 0.5 being a moderate change, and approximately 0.8 being a large change.[12] Norman suggested that a reasonable estimate of an MCID corresponds to an effect size of 0.5.[13,14]

In the publication of the van Rijssen and associates' 6-week RCT results,[15] the disabilities of the arm, shoulder and hand (DASH) questionnaire is used as secondary outcome. The DASH is a validated, patient-reported outcome measure. It is a questionnaire that consists of 30 items and is scored from 0 to 100. In this scale, a lower score means the patient experiences less disability. In general, for hand function, the DASH has an MCID of 10.[16–18] This means it would take a decrease in DASH score of 10 for a patient to perceive a benefit from their treatment. The value of the MCID is not shared with the reader in the 6-week RCT results.[15] Therefore, although the reader is told that "DASH scores of both groups differed significantly at all time points after treatment," the reader cannot be sure whether this difference in DASH score was clinically significant for the patient.

IMPORTANT CONCEPTS IN APPLYING RESULTS TO PATIENT CARE
Can the Results be Applied to My Patient?

The patient sitting in your office will often have different characteristics than the patients who were enrolled in the trial. Your patient may be older or younger, with or without comorbidity or other demographic factors that would have excluded them from participation in the trial.

If inclusion and exclusion criteria are clearly reported in the trial manuscript and your patient meets the inclusion criteria, without violating the exclusion criteria, you can confidently apply the results to your patient. The authors' patient, Mr White, fits the inclusion criteria and would not have been excluded from this trial (**Box 3**).

However, what if the patient sitting in your office does not meet the study inclusion criteria? The results of a trial would likely still apply to your patient if, for example, he/she has a comorbidity, or is 4 years too old to have been included in the trial. A good approach to decide whether the results can be applied to your patient is to ask whether there is a compelling reason the results should not apply to your patient.[3]

On the other hand, treatments, especially surgical interventions, may not be uniformly effective. Because the results of an RCT are an estimate of the average treatment effect, applying this average effect means the surgeon may expose the patient who may only benefit slightly from the surgery, to the full cost or risk of the intervention.[4]

Were All Clinically Important Outcomes Considered?

Treatments are indicated when they provide important benefits.[3] Hand surgeons should use appropriate techniques to measure relevant

---

Box 3
Inclusion and exclusion criteria of the RCT: LF versus PNF

Inclusion Criteria

1. A flexion contracture of at least 30° in the metacarpophalangeal, proximal interphalangeal, or distal interphalangeal joints

2. A clearly defined pathologic cord in the palmar fascia

3. Willingness to participate in this trial

Exclusion Criteria

1. Patients with post-surgical recurrence or extension of the disease

2. Patients who were not allowed to stop taking their anticoagulants

3. Patients generally unfit to have surgery

4. Patients who were not willing to participate in this study or had a specific treatment wish

Data from van Rijssen AL, Gerbrandy FS, ter Linden H, et al. A comparison of the direct outcomes of percutaneous needle fasciotomy and limited fasciectomy for Dupuytren's disease: a 6-week follow-up study. J Hand Surg Am 2006;31:717–25.

endpoints. This objective should be balanced with the potential of burdening patients with several assessments and questionnaires.

Physical tests and biomechanical measurements (ie, range of motion, pinch strength, grip strength etc.) are the most commonly reported outcome measures in hand surgery.[19] Although objective and reproducible measurements can be obtained, these outcomes may not reflect the true benefit of a treatment to the patient. What the surgeon might view as a considerable improvement in grip strength may not correspond to improved hand function from the patient's perspective.[20]

Both patients and clinicians should use a measurement that demonstrates the intervention improves the outcome that is important to the patient, *patient-important outcomes*. The interest in *patient-important outcomes*, and the shift away from objective, physical measures, has lead to an increase in health-related quality of life (HRQL) questionnaires.[19] These patient-reported questionnaires are either broad, general health questionnaires or region-specific and disease-specific questionnaires. Some examples of validated patient-reported questionnaires in hand surgery are listed in **Box 4**.

When examined closely, the primary outcome of the van Rijssen and associates' RCT[6] is information from a continuous biomechanical measurement (degrees of joint contracture) abridged into a dichotomous outcome of recurrence (contracture >30° or <30°). Using a validated scale such as the DASH,[21] QuickDASH, MHQ,[22] or the more recent Health Utilities Index (HUI, a generic

quality of life scale from which utilities can be calculated)[24] could have been more useful in interpreting the benefit of the procedures. The MHQ and the HUI-3 have been shown to be reliable and valid tools when assessing patients with Dupuytren disease.[25] A new scale, specific to Dupuytren contracture will be useful for future hand surgery trials. The Unité Rhumatologique des Affections de la Main (URAM) is a practical 9-item scale with a scoring system of 0 to 45, which has also been validated for Dupuytren disease.[26] This scale was not available when van Rijssen and colleagues started their study.

Are the Likely Treatment Benefits Worth the Potential Harm?

The final step in interpreting the effectiveness of a treatment is to decide whether the benefits of the intervention are worth the effort and risk that you and the patient will invest in the treatment and post-operative recovery. As discussed earlier, a large RRR may appear impressive, although the impact on your patient could be minimal. The concept of NNT can be used to examine the absolute impact of the intervention on your practice. The NNT is the inverse of the *ARR* (NNT = 1/ARR).

In the van Rijssen and associates' RCT (van Rijssen 2012), for the primary outcome of 5-year recurrence, the NNT = 1/0.616 = 1.6, or 2. This suggests that for every 2 patients treated with LF, as opposed to PNF, the surgeon can prevent one episode of recurrence.

Infections were rare in the van Rijssen and associates' RCT.[6] When evaluated at 1 week, the

Box 4
Commonly used patient-reported outcome instruments in hand surgery

Instrument	Relevant Health Condition	Scoring of Scale
Michigan Hand Questionnaire (MHQ)	Various health states related to hand disorders	• 37-item scale • Total score 0–100
Disabilities of the Arm, Shoulder and Hand Questionnaire (DASH)	Upper extremity physical function and symptoms	• 30-item scale • Total score 0–100
Quick Disabilities of the Arm, Shoulder and Hand Questionnaire (QuickDASH)	Upper extremity physical function and symptoms	• 11-item scale • Total score 0–100
Carpal Tunnel Questionnaire (Boston Questionnaire)	Severity of symptoms, and functional status related to carpal tunnel syndrome	• Symptom severity scale, 11-items • Functional severity scale, 8-itmes

Data from Refs.[21–23]

infection rate for the LF group was 1.8% and in the PNF group was 0%. The *absolute risk difference* for infection at 1 week was ARR = 1.8% − 0% = 1.8%. The number needed to harm (NNH) (where NNH is the number of interventions needed to harm one additional patient) would be NNH = 1/ARR = 1/0.018 = 55.6, or 56 patients.

Therefore, for every 100 patients we consider treating with LF, we would expect to prevent 50 episodes of recurrence (NNT = 2, 100/2 = 50), at the cost of having 2 infections (NNH = 56, 100/56 = 1.79, or 2). When considering this information, the utility of LF in Dupuytren disease becomes more certain. Understanding the concept of NNT and NNH for relevant events helps the surgeon and patient weigh the benefits against potential harms associated with the intervention.

Are the Likely Treatment Benefits Worth the Potential Costs?

Hand surgeons are now expected both to use the best available evidence to guide clinical decisions and to ensure that the treatment will be cost-effective. Collecting cost data simultaneously while executing an RCT allows investigators to piggyback an economic evaluation to the trial.[27]

Important steps in performing an economic analysis include deciding which costs (direct or indirect) and consequences (a single outcome like recurrence or a patient-important outcome measure like the DASH) to be measured. Furthermore, a decision must be made on which economic perspective to take: the Patient, a Hospital/Clinical Practice, a Third Party Payer (like Medicare or the National Health Service), or Society. Guidelines on conducting and interpreting the results of an economic evaluation in plastic and hand surgery are available.[27–29]

An economic evaluation was not performed in the van Rijssen and associates' RCT.[6] Only 95 economic evaluations comparing 2 plastic surgery interventions have been published between 1986 and 2012; 79% of these evaluations were found to be only partial economic evaluations (cost analyses).[30] In a systematic review of hand surgery studies, Chung and colleagues[31] identified a specific need for more research on economic analysis. Therefore, in an era of diminishing health care resources, there is an opportunity to incorporate economic evaluations into surgical clinical research and contain health care costs.

SUMMARY

Results of surgical interventions are viewed as highly variable due to known and unknown patient factors, as well as differences in preoperative care,

post-operative care, and surgeon technique and experience. When interpreting the results of a trial, it is important to perform a methodical assessment to determine whether a study is providing valid results and how these results can be applied in your patient's clinical context. Although clinicians perform this general process when discussing the risks and benefits of a therapy with their patient, the ability to interpret and understand the strength of the available evidence is essential. This process will help surgeons incorporate evidence-based surgery into their practice and improve patient care.

REFERENCES

1. Evidence-Based Medicine Working Group. Evidence-based medicine. A new approach to the teaching of medicine. JAMA 1992;268(17):2420–5.
2. Waljee J, Larson BP, Chung KC. Measuring treatment effectiveness: a guide to incorporating the principles of evidence-based medicine. Plast Reconstr Surg 2012;130(6):1382–94.
3. Guyatt G, Rennie D, Meade M, et al. Users' guides to the medical literature: a manual for evidence-based clinical practice. 2nd edition. New York: McGraw-Hill; 2008.
4. Bhandari M, Haynes RH. How to appraise the effectiveness of treatment. World J Surg 2005;29:570–5.
5. Graham B. Strategies for nonrandomized clinical research in hand surgery. Clin Plast Surg 2005;32:529–36.
6. van Rijssen AL, ter Linden H, Werker PM. Five-year results of a randomized clinical trial on treatment in Dupuytren's disease: percutaneous needle fasciotomy versus limited fasciectomy. Plast Reconstr Surg 2012;129(2):467–77.
7. Thoma A, Farrokhyar F, Bhandari M, et al. Users' guide to the surgical literature how to assess a randomized controlled trial in surgery. Can J Surg 2004;47(3):200–8.
8. Thoma A. Challenges in creating a good randomized controlled trial in hand surgery. Clin Plast Surg 2005;32:563–73.
9. Cadeddu M, Farrokhyar F, Levis C, et al, for the Evidence-Based Surgery Working Group. Users' guide to the surgical literature: understanding confidence intervals. Can J Surg 2012;55(3):207–11.
10. Jaeschke R, Singer J, Guyatt GH. Ascertaining the minimal clinically important difference. Control Clin Trials 1989;10:407–15.
11. Cadeddu M, Farrokhyar F, Thoma A, et al, for the Evidence-Based Surgery Working Group. Users' guide to the surgical literature: how to assess power and sample size. Can J Surg 2008;51(6):476–82.
12. Cohen J. Statistical power analysis in the behavioural sciences. Hillsdale (NJ): Erlbaum; 1988.

13. Norman GR, Sridhar FG, Guyatt GH, et al. Relation of distribution and anchor-based approaches in interpretation of changes in health-related quality of life. Med Care 2001;39(10):1039–47.

14. Norman GR, Sloan JA, Wyrwich KW. Interpretation of changes in health-related quality of life: the remarkable universality of half a standard deviation. Med Care 2003;41(5):582–92.

15. van Rijssen AL, Gerbrandy FS, ter Linden H, et al. A comparison of the direct outcomes of percutaneous needle fasciotomy and limited fasciectomy for Dupuytren's disease: a 6-week follow-up study. J Hand Surg Am 2006;31:717–25.

16. Beaton DE, Davis AM, Hudak P, et al. The DASH (disabilities of the arm, shoulder and hand) outcome measure: what do we know about it now? Br J Hand Ther 2001;6(4):109–18.

17. Hunsaker FG, Cioffi DA, Amadio PC, et al. The American academy of orthopaedic surgeons outcomes instruments: normative values from the general population. J Bone Joint Surg Am 2002;84(2):208–15.

18. Beaton DE, van Eerd D, Smith P, et al. Minimal change is sensitive, less specific to recovery: a diagnostic testing approach to interpretability. J Clin Epidemiol 2011;64(5):487–96.

19. Alderman AK, Chung KC. Measuring outcomes in hand surgery. Clin Plast Surg 2008;35:239–50.

20. Giladi AM, Chung KC. Measuring outcomes in hand surgery. Clin Plast Surg 2013;40:313–22.

21. Hudak PL, Amadio PC, Bombardier C. Development of an upper extremity outcome measure: the DASH (Disabilities of the Arm, Shoulder, and Head). Am J Ind Med 1996;29:602–8.

22. Chung KC, Pillsbury MS, Walters MR, et al. Reliability and validity testing of the Michigan Hand Outcomes Questionnaire. J Hand Surg Am 1998;23(4):575–87.

23. Levine DW, Simmons BP, Koris MJ, et al. A self-administered questionnaire for the assessment of severity of symptoms and functional status in carpal tunnel syndrome. J Bone Joint Surg Am 1993;75(11):1585–92.

24. Furlong WJ, Feeny DH, Torrance GW, et al. The Health Utilities Index (HUI) system for assessing health-related quality of life in clinical studies. Ann Med 2001;33(5):375–84.

25. Thoma A, Kaur MN, Ignacy TA, et al. Psychometric properties of health related quality of life instruments in patients undergoing palmar fasciectomy for Dupuytren's disease: a prospective study. Hand 2014;9(2):166–74.

26. Beaudreuil J, Allard A, Zerkak D, et al, URAM Study Group. Unité Rhumatologique des Affections de la Main (URAM) scale: development and validation of a tool to assess Dupuytren's disease-specific disability. Arthritis Care Res (Hoboken) 2011;63(10):1448–55.

27. Thoma A, Sprague S, Tandan V. Users' guide to the surgical literature: how to use an article on economic analysis. Can J Surg 2001;44(5):347–54.

28. Thoma A, Strumas N, Rockwell G, et al. The use of cost-effectiveness analysis in plastic surgery clinical research. Clin Plast Surg 2008;35:2850296.

29. Kotsis SV, Chung KC. Fundamental principles of conducting a surgery economic analysis study. Plast Reconstr Surg 2010;125:727–35.

30. Ziolkowski NI, Voineskos SH, Ignacy TA, et al. Systematic review of economic evaluations in plastic surgery [systematic review]. Plast Reconstr Surg 2013;132(1):191–203.

31. Chung KC, Burns PB, Sears ED. Outcomes research in hand surgery: where have we been and where should we go? J Hand Surg Am 2006;31:1373–9.

Patient-Reported Outcomes

State-of-the-Art Hand Surgery and Future Applications

Joy C. MacDermid, BScPT, PhD[a,b,*]

KEYWORDS

- Patient-reported outcome measures • Hand surgery • Upper extremity

KEY POINTS

- A key element of the selection of patient-reported outcome measures (PRO) is understanding the content/conceptual domain covered by different options, and matching these to the population and purpose.
- The Numeric Pain Rating Scale, Michigan Hand Questionnaire, Patient-Rated Wrist (Hand) Evaluation, and Disabilities of the Arm, Shoulder, Hand questionnaire are reliable and valid outcome measures for hand conditions.
- Ideally measures should have interval-level scaling, a wide range of measurement capacity, consistent responses when patients are stable, and responsiveness when patients change, and should have formal validation for other cultures/languages.
- Differential item functioning, response bias, ceiling/floor effects, literacy issues, and other factors can result in failure to achieve accurate measurement with PRO.

Patient-reported outcome measures (PRO), once considered subjective and unreliable, are now recognized as pivotal to understanding the impact of clinical decisions. The 5 steps of evidence-based practice (**Box 1**) require moving from specific clinical questions generated on the basis of interaction with a patient, to finding and applying the best available clinical research evidence—in combination with clinical expertise and patient values and preferences—to make the optimal patient-centered, evidence-informed decision.[1,2] The next step in the process of becoming an evidence-based practitioner is to evaluate the outcomes of evidence-informed decisions.[3] Given that evidence-based practice is designed to incorporate patient values and preferences in decision making,[4–7] the outcome of that decision from the perspective of the patient is central to our effectiveness as evidence-based practitioners.

Increasingly it has become recognized that new drugs, devices, and other interventions must prove themselves in terms of better outcomes at the patient level to warrant investment of public or private dollars. Over the past decade, the Food and Drug Administration has moved toward creating standards of expectation on proving better patient outcomes when approving new drugs and devices.[8] The research community has recognized the importance of PRO, in that most large trials now use PRO as the primary outcome of interest to determine the effectiveness of interventions. The importance of PRO is acknowledged by

[a] School of Rehabilitation Sciences, McMaster University, IAHS, 1400 Main Street West, 4th Floor, Hamilton, Ontario L8S 1C7, Canada; [b] Clinical Research Laboratory, Hand and Upper Limb Centre, St. Joseph's Health Centre, London, 268 Grosvenor Street, Ontario N6A 4L6, Canada
* School of Rehabilitation Science, IAHS, 1400 Main Street West, 4th Floor, Hamilton, Ontario L8S 1C7, Canada.
E-mail address: macderj@mcmaster.ca

Hand Clin 30 (2014) 293–304
http://dx.doi.org/10.1016/j.hcl.2014.04.003
0749-0712/14/$ – see front matter © 2014 Elsevier Inc. All rights reserved.

indicate that use of PRO by therapists is low in many musculoskeletal upper extremity conditions,[9–13] despite pain and disability being the predominant complaints. Although the use of PRO by physicians is rarely reported, the limited evidence indicates it is substantially lower than use by therapists.[11] There has been a rapid increase in the use of PRO in clinical trials, which is likely related to regulator and funding agency pressures requiring that interventions demonstrate effectiveness for patient outcomes.[8] Most clinical trials use a PRO as their primary outcome, with impairment and imaging considered as secondary measures. However, when it comes to clinical practice the reverse is often true. Substantial implementation of PRO in clinical practice where insurers mandate their use is now becoming apparent. In interviews with clinicians one often finds that PRO are implemented because they are required, but that they are not consistently used in decision making. Situations whereby outcome measures are selected simply to satisfy the needs of insurers represent a substantial lost opportunity. The potential value of PRO in clinical decision making is sizable. However, unless clinicians select outcome measures thoughtfully, they may not be a valid representation of the patient's status, treatment effects, or outcomes (**Box 2**).

professional groups, including hand surgeons and hand therapists, although implementation has been less speedy in the clinical arena than in the research arena.

IMPLEMENTATION OF OUTCOME MEASURES

Despite the great advances in the development of reliable and valid PRO, the implementation process has been slow, which is not surprising as there is always a lag between invention and implementation, typically up to 10 to 20 years in many areas of medicine. Practice pattern studies

MEASURING PRO: CONTENT DOMAIN

It is important to consider the construct or content domain measured by a tool when evaluating its appropriateness for any specific measurement purpose or context. PRO, like any other measurement tool, will have specific measurement properties in terms of what they are capable of measuring, the range and precision that can be measured, and the factors that will invalidate accurate measurement. Some outcome measures are designed to measure broad concepts, such as quality of life, that involve personal interpretation of one's circumstances and how one's expectations are met.[14–16] It must be expected that two individuals with identical upper extremity problems would have very different ratings of quality of life depending on their individual circumstances, including health concerns beyond their upper extremity problems. Health-related quality of life focuses on satisfaction with life circumstances in the context of health. Health status focuses on specific domains of health, and is intended to encompass a broad view of health that applies to most individuals. These terms, though sometimes used interchangeably, represent different conceptual domains.

MEASURING PRO: GENERIC VERSUS CONDITION-SPECIFIC INSTRUMENTS

Because upper extremity surgery and rehabilitation focuses on restoring the function of the upper limb, there is often concern that generic health status or quality-of-life instruments do not pick up the concerns and treatment responses that are salient to this population. More specific instruments include the regional instruments such as the Disabilities of the Arm, Shoulder, Hand[17,18] (DASH), which focuses on the function of the upper extremity, and joint-specific measures such as the Patient-Rated Wrist Evaluation (PRWE)[19–21] or the Simple Shoulder Test,[22,23] designed to focus on symptoms and functional limitations arising from health conditions affecting a body area. Other measures are condition specific, such as the Symptom Severity Scale[24] designed for carpal tunnel syndrome. Condition-specific measures are most relevant when there are unusual features or a specific cluster of symptoms/impairments that would not be captured by generic tools. For example, it might be argued that carpal tunnel syndrome and shoulder instability are sufficiently unique conditions that they are not well served by more generic measures. The need for a generic or specific scale can be determined through clinical measurement studies. Measures can also

focus on a specific symptom, such as the McGill Pain Questionnaire[25,26] and the Pain Catastrophizing Scale,[27,28] or can measure a specific participation, such as the Work Instability Scale.[29–32] An instrument must demonstrate content validity; that is, its items and instructions must capture the concept that it proposes to measure. This aspect is perhaps the most fundamental one in measurement validity, but is often poorly addressed. Therefore, it is important that end users clearly understand the conceptual domain that an instrument has been designed to measure.

Most measures are provided in a format whereby preset, standardized questions are presented to the respondents. However, some patient-specific measures are devised to allow the respondents to select the items that are of importance to them, and to respond to these on a common metric. The Canadian Occupational Performance Measure (COPM)[33–36] and the Patient-Specific Functional Scale[37–39] are measures of this type, and have been used in a variety of conditions, including hand disorders.[34,38,40,41] The benefit of these measures is that they are more patient centered; the downside is that scores are not comparable across patients because the items are not standardized and have not been calibrated to a specific level of difficulty.

MEASURING PRO: ADMINISTRATION FORMAT

PRO are most commonly administered as a paper-based questionnaire. Some instruments are meant to be verbally administered, such as the COPM[36] or the verbal numeric pain rating scale.[42] Many PRO, including the DASH,[43] have been validated to be administered verbally (ie, over the phone), or in some cases by surrogate respondents. This transferability of PRO to different administration methods allows clinicians and researchers to collect more comprehensive outcomes information. Many of these paper-based instruments have now been developed for electronic formats to be administered through the Web or applications. The most recent developments in administration of PRO have increasingly relied on technology, such as those involved with apps or computer-adaptive testing (CAT).

Examples of PRO relevant to hand surgery are listed in **Table 1**.

ADVANTAGES AND LIMITATIONS IN USING PRO IN CLINICAL RESEARCH

The most important advantage of PRO in clinical research is that they can provide standardized

Table 1
Examples of PRO relevant to hand surgery

Construct (Type of PRO)	Examples
Pain (symptom specific)	Numeric Pain Rating Scale[42] Visual Analog Scale[42,44,45] McGill Pain Questionnaire[25,26,46–49] Pain subscale of the Patient-Rated Wrist Evaluation (PRWE)[19,21,50]; Patient-Rated Elbow Evaluation (PREE)[51]; Patient-Rated Tennis Elbow Evaluation (PRTEE)[52]; Patient-Rated Ulnar Nerve Evaluation (PRUNE)[53]
Psychosocial aspects or impact of pain	Pain Catastrophizing Scale[27,54] Pain Interference Scale[42]
Symptoms for specific upper extremity conditions (condition specific)	Symptom Severity Scale (carpal tunnel syndrome)[24] AusCan pain and stiffness subscales (hand osteoarthritis)[55,56] Tennis elbow (PRTEE)[52,57]
Function for specific upper extremity conditions (condition specific)	AusCan function subscale (hand osteoarthritis)[55,56] Function subscale of carpal tunnel instrument[24] Shoulder instability[58]
Function of the upper extremity (regional)	Disabilities of the Arm, Shoulder, Hand (DASH)[17,18] or QuickDASH[59] Upper Extremity Functional Index[60] Upper Extremity Functional Scale[61]
Function of a specific upper extremity joint or joint complex ("joint" specific)	PRW(H)E[19,20,50] Michigan Hand Questionnaire (MHQ)[62–64] PREE[51] American Shoulder and Elbow Surgeons (ASES)—elbow[65] Shoulder Pain and Disability Index (SPADI)[66,67] ASES—shoulder[22] Simple Shoulder Test[68,69]
Work disability (participation specific)	Work Limitations Questionnaire[70–72] Work Instability Scale[29,30,32,73]
Physical activity (participation specific)	Rapid Assessment of Physical Activity (RAPA)[74,75]
Quality of life for specific upper extremity conditions (condition-specific quality of life)	Western Ontario Rotator Cuff (WORC)[76] Western Ontario Osteoarthritis Shoulder (WOOS)[77]
Patient-Specific Measure	Patient-Specific Functional Scale[37] Canadian Occupational Performance Measure[34–36,78]

measures indicating whether the patient is better off after an intervention. In the past, clinical research studies often focused on impairment measures, such as radiographic alignment or grip strength, which may not have captured the patient's perspective. Furthermore, PRO can capture multiple domains to better assess the nature of the impact of the intervention. PRO can simplify the difficult task of conducting trials across multiple centers because they provide a standardized outcome that can be obtained across multiple sites without requiring substantial standardization of equipment and training across sites.

Challenges in using PRO in clinical research exist. It may require multiple measures to capture all of the impacts of importance in musculoskeletal disability, as these conditions tend to affect many domains of life. Administering multiple measures can create a substantial patient burden. Because most PRO are developed in English, when conducting multicenter trials it is only possible for non-English sites to participate if they have access to appropriate cross-cultural translations. Cross-cultural translation research is an important aspect of clinical measurement science, but can be difficult to fund or publish. Formal cross-cultural translation is essential to inclusiveness in measurement. Furthermore, cross-cultural translation research helps clinicians to better understand how PRO work in different populations and increase the pool of comparative data. Although there has been a vast proliferation in the development of PRO, not all clinically relevant concepts have been addressed. Hence, researchers may not find a measure appropriate to their purpose or population.

In other cases, there are multiple PRO that address the same conceptual domain, and there is no evidence to suggest superiority. For example, the DASH, PRWE, and Michigan Hand Questionnaire (MHQ) all have empirical support. In clinical research, responsiveness to detect change is a critical issue in selecting an outcome measure because it will be a primary determinant of the sample size required to detect treatment effectiveness. Therefore, studies of responsiveness in the specific population and intervention may be needed to establish the optimal trial protocol. PRO are able to measure change over a specific range, so they may not be responsive for certain patients who would benefit from an intervention. For example, patients who have very high function, such as athletes or injured workers, may be able to perform all of the activities on commonly used upper extremity PRO. However, the scale may not be capable of detecting the substantial loss of ability for these high-functioning patients. Conversely, patients at very low levels of function such as those in nursing homes may not perform any of the activities listed on PRO, which often assume that people are living independently. Important impacts of improved hand function in mobility, dressing, and eating may not be reflected in these instruments. These problems are often termed floor-and-ceiling effects. When such patients are included in trials, the instrument may not measure the effectiveness of the treatment in those participants. In general, when designing a trial the inclusion/exclusion criteria should consider defining who is potentially responsive to the intervention, and whether their improvement could be measured by the selected instruments. For example, in some pain trials it is specified that patients must have pain that is at least 4/10 on a numeric pain rating to be included. Including patients in a trial where the outcome measures will not be responsive reduces power. Finally, many PRO have not been shown to demonstrate interval-level scaling, but rather are in fact ordinal measures. However, many trials analyze the scores with parametric statistics appropriate for interval-level measurement, rather than nonparametric statistics that should be used with ordinal data.

ADVANTAGES AND LIMITATIONS IN USING PRO IN CLINICAL PRACTICE

A primary advantage of using PRO is that they are patient centered. Patients appreciate that their view is considered in evaluating the impact of care and regularly monitoring their progress.[79] Many of the items reflect important concepts that clinicians would typically inquire about in their patient histories. Standardized data collection of the patients' perspective on their status provides feedback to the clinician about the extent and nature of improvements that occur with intervention. These data can provide guideposts for when progress is stalled, or when patients reach important milestones that might support discharge. PRO can be important predictors of future outcomes. Studies have shown that return to work following distal radius fractures is better predicted by the PRWE than by a battery of impairment measures including grip, range of motion, and dexterity.[80] PRO can also identify patients with poor prognosis who may need particular modifications to their intervention plan. For example, patients with high levels of pain or pain catastrophizing have been shown to be at higher risk of persistent pain and disability.[81–83] Patient and clinician burden being an important consideration, many valid PRO measurement tools take 5 minutes or less to complete and can efficiently fit into a typical practice setting. Although few studies address how PRO affect practice, there is limited evidence suggesting that incorporating PRO improves dimensions of practice.[78]

There are also challenges in incorporating measures into clinical practice. Whereas having many different PRO in one's clinic can be challenging, having only one is unlikely to meet the needs of all patients. The range of issues already discussed is even more critical when applying measures to individual patients. Most PRO assess function by asking about tasks of daily life, and may not capture substantial loss of function in patients who have either very high or low levels of function. When these measures are used to assess the need for surgery or therapy, care might be denied because the instrument is not picking up important deficits. The best solution for this in clinical practice is to use a patient-specific measure whereby the individual picks items that are particularly salient to his or her health problem.

There are also substantial and vastly underestimated barriers for patients with literacy difficulty.[84,85] Measures should be designed at grade 6 reading level, and the readability and clarity of PRO instruments must be thoroughly assessed before they are published in the literature. Cognitive interviewing[86,87] is a technique that can be used to assess how potential respondents understand, interpret, and calibrate items on PRO measurement instruments. However, this technique has only recently been gaining widespread usage. Some patients may be literate in their native language but not in English. Unless there are appropriate cross-cultural translations of PRO, some patients may be excluded from assessment procedures on this basis. Hence, clinicians often find once they implement PRO that they will have a subset of patients for whom the tool is not a valid measure of status for any of the aforestated reasons.

PRO scores can also be difficult for clinicians and patients to interpret, and many continue to rely on their impairment measures. Familiarity with the trajectory of recovery and expected scores for different conditions over time will evolve as clinicians gain experience with a PRO instrument. Many clinicians tend to forget that they did not intuitively know the appropriate range of motion for a postoperative flexor tendon repair until they had substantial experience measuring range of motion in that particular patient population. Thus, clinicians often develop the same intuition about whether patients are presenting a typical score as they continue to use PRO in practice. PRO provide a unique perspective on objective, functional measures, and can augment the understanding of recovery. For example, a functional impairment measure, such as grip strength, may improve over time, with no improvement in self-reported disability or pain. It is possible that the instrument used to measure this concept is not responsive for the type of patient being evaluated, so that a different PRO instrument is needed. However, it may also be that the impairment is improving but is not an important determinant of patient functioning, so that the clinician needs to reconsider the focus of treatment. Finally, a disconnection between impairment and disability indicates that psychosocial or environmental factors are playing a substantial role in the disablement process. Clinicians need to become familiar with the strategies for ensuring that they know how to interpret the meaning of a PRO score for an individual patient (**Box 3**).

APPROACHES TO APPLYING OUTCOME MEASURE SCORES TO INDIVIDUAL PATIENTS

The first step in measuring patients is to ensure that due diligence has been performed to select an outcome measure that has established reliability and validity, and measures the constructs relevant to the individual patient. Ideally the instrument should be able to provide interval-level

---

Box 3
Information needed to interpret PRO in individual patients

1. Does the selected PRO and associated scoring algorithm provide interval-level measurement?

2. Are there normative scores?

3. Are there comparative scores for different clinical populations at different time points that might be used for establishing benchmarks or comparisons?

4. What is the measurement error expected for a single measurement at one point in time (MDC)?

5. How responsive is the instrument to picking up change that can occur either with improvement or decline? How does this compare with other instruments that measure the same concept?

6. What is the range over which this instrument will provide a valid assessment of status and allow for measurement of change?

7. How much change is required to indicate that the patient has experienced a CID?

---

scoring as indicated by Rasch analysis. Some instruments have Rasch-based scoring algorithms that were published after original development, this being is a more recent technique. Without this, clinicians should be cautious about expecting the clinically important difference (CID) or minimal detectable change (MDC) to apply equally across the entire range of the scale.

Several PRO instruments will have normative scores published. Although this can be useful information, clinicians must be cautious in assuming that once patients reach "normal range for your age" they will be satisfied with their outcome. Musculoskeletal disability is known to increase with age; hence, normative scores reflect the prevalence of musculoskeletal disability in the population. Normative scores can be useful for research applications, but are typically less useful in clinical practice. Individual patients are typically more concerned with regaining their preinjury level of functioning than whether they are equivalent to their age-matched peers. More useful is to have comparative data on the expected rate of recovery after surgical interventions or injuries. Compiling comparative information at different time points and interventions in patient cohorts can provide useful comparative data for clinicians and researchers when writing reports. Some studies have published growth curves to describe these recovery trajectories. It can be useful in clinical practice to show patients whether they are on a typical trajectory or not. Clinicians should be aware of whether the PRO they are using is able to pick up change for a specific patient population, and consider whether it is relevant for each patient they evaluate. Information about responsiveness is commonly reported in the literature. When an instrument seems to be demonstrating problems related to range (ceiling or floor effects), an alternative such as the Patient-Specific Functional Scale can be used to improve evaluation for specific patients.

Substantial attention in the clinical measurement literature has been given to the development of criteria for evaluating change in PRO. The MDC is based on the reliability of the measure and the variability in the underlying population, and provides an indicator of how much change must occur to be confident (usually 90% confidence) that the score has changed beyond what might be expected by chance. Usually, clinicians should expect to see this amount of change in a relatively short time if PRO is to be useful in indicating change in patient status. For example, the MDC for the DASH and PRWE has been estimated to be approximately 10 points. Naturally, this varies according to the population studied. However, the MDC is often used to set short-term goals. The minimal CID is determined based on several different analytical techniques that are designed to determine how much change is clinically meaningful. This concept reflects the change that a clinician should expect to ensure treatment benefit (and should be considered when setting long-term goals). Again, the caveat for MDC and CID is that these assume that interval-level measurement is present. It is commonly considered that 2 points is a CID on a numeric rating scale.[88] Where CID is missing, 20% can be a useful approximate indicator of important difference. Comparative data are also important for setting goals. For example, when patients were divided into groups who were able to work versus being unable to work, this was reflected by DASH scores in the 20s versus 50s.[17]

RECENT INNOVATIONS IN OUTCOME MEASUREMENT
Evolution of Clinical Measurement as a Science

Clinical measurement science is a field with rapidly evolving methodologies. Experts in developing and evaluating PRO have specialized methodological expertise in the same way that clinical trialists do. Earlier clinical measurement science had

a substantial focus on classic psychometric/clinimetric methods that provided information about measurement properties such as reliability, different forms of validity, and responsiveness. More modern methods often focus on mathematical models (Rasch model, item response theory) that assume PRO should be able to measure latent traits.[89,90] These methods allow researchers to evaluate existing measurement tools using new indicators of item functioning, unidimensionality, differential item functioning, and interval-level scaling. More rigorous methods in assessing the content of outcome measures have developed through the International Classification of Functioning, Disability and Health (ICF) linking,[91] cognitive interviewing, and other techniques that place greater focus on ensuring the conceptual validity of PRO.

Interval-level scaling is a critical feature of PRO because it is important that "the ruler" behaves the same way throughout its range. Failure to achieve interval-level scaling has been demonstrated for several PRO. This finding is understandable because many PRO were developed using clinimetric methods, which did not lend themselves to this type of evaluation. However, commonly used indicators such as MDC and CID are not meaningful if a change score does not apply equally across different aspects of the scale. If certain subgroups of patients answer questions differently (differential item functioning), this can contaminate the conclusions about treatment effectiveness. Fortunately, many of the existing measures can be "rescued" by providing alternative scoring algorithms or revised scales. There has been a recent proliferation of such studies. The challenge now is when to place a new or revised measure in the public domain. Because it can take a substantial effort to move a PRO into practice and to collect a useful pool of comparative data, the benefit of a new PRO must be clear.

Development of Core Sets of Content Related to Hand Function

Many PRO used in hand surgery focus on function. The international standard for classifying function is the ICF.[92–94] This classification system consists of many different codes structured in a hierarchical system and designed to provide a common language by which one can describe how a person functions in society. The establishment of core sets for different health conditions is a rigorous process through which the international community meets and reviews research in the area, patient data, and expert opinion, to conduct consensus exercises that result in a small subset of

ICF codes that are most relevant to describing people with a specific health condition.[95–97] As such, these represent a gold standard of the important domains that apply for specific health conditions. The establishment of core sets for hand conditions (http://www.icf-research-branch.org/icf-core-sets-projects-sp-1641024398/other-health-conditions/development-of-icf-core-sets-for-hand-conditions) provides a valuable resource for clinicians, researchers, and policymakers to communicate internationally using a common language. ICF codes, including the core sets, provide a structure and rigorous method for comparing content, and represent a substantial advance in content validation over less rigorous methods such as expert review or face validity.

Consensus on Core Constructs

With the development of multiple PRO and increased awareness of their importance, there has been a move to have international discussions and consensus exercises that focus on what clinicians should be measuring. For example, the international community recently reflected on the use of outcome measures in distal radius fracture through evidence reviews, followed by workshops and consensus exercises sponsored by the International Society for Fracture Repair and The International Osteoporosis Foundation. The goal was to make consensus recommendations about the use of outcome measures for evaluation in this patient population.[98] This group recommended that pain and function should be measured separately, and that simple measures that could be used in everyday practice include a numeric pain rating or the PRWE pain subscale, and the QuickDASH or PRWE function subscale. Radiology and impairment measures were considered secondary outcomes, while recognizing that they can be important in guiding treatment but are less directly relevant as outcome indicators.

The National Institutes of Health (NIH) recently sponsored a large "toolbox" effort (http://www.nihtoolbox.org/Pages/default.aspx) to establish core measures for clinical research. The NIH toolbox recommendations for pain included, at minimum, a numeric pain rating scale and a pain interference scale.[42] The NIH also established the Patient Reported Outcomes Measurement Information System (PROMIS) to promote high-quality common data element instruments by which PRO can be measured and compared across conditions (http://www.nihtoolbox.org/Pages/default.aspx).

It is appropriate that when consensus exercises are conducted they are viewed as guidelines. There are many mediating factors relevant to why different outcome measures may be used in different situations. Furthermore, using clinical measurement techniques, one should be able to establish metrics to translate scores onto a common metric. Meta-analyses often include concepts that are measured with different tools to provide more complete inclusion of all available research in estimates of intervention effects.

Computerized Forms of PRO

Traditionally, many PRO were administered by paper-based questionnaires. In fact, this continues to be the practice in many hand surgery and hand therapy clinics. However, with the proliferation of electronic medical records and highly portable personal computing devices, it is becoming feasible to administer PRO electronically. For example, there is an app that can be used to administer the DASH (http://www.dash.iwh.on.ca/app); there are Web sites that provide the questions and scoring algorithms for many orthopedic PRO (http://www.orthopaedicscore.com/); and there are multiple electronic medical record systems that incorporate PRO within the software. All of these have increased accessibility of administration and improved usefulness of PRO, because it is now easier to track changes over time. Despite this, there are still many small hand surgery practices and clinics providing much of the care for people with hand conditions where electronic medical systems may be cost prohibitive. The availability of low-cost apps provides an option whereby infrastructure is less supersized. With any new method of collecting patient information, there is always a need to ensure data security and confidentiality.

Web sites for commonly used hand questionnaires

DASH: http://www.dash.iwh.on.ca/

PRWE (and related measures): http://www.srs-mcmaster.ca/Default.aspx?tabid=3784

MHQ: http://sitemaker.umich.edu/mhq/mhq

Computer-Adaptive Testing

One of the most common concerns in clinical research is the patient burden of administering questionnaires. Researchers are often interested in multiple domains to determine whether an intervention is effective, and what specific health domains are affected. This approach requires multiple measures to be administered across multiple time points. The more items there are on a questionnaire, the more reliable it tends to be. When administering standardized PRO everyone must answer the same set of questions, so there will often be questions that are too difficult or too easy for any given patient based on the level of health. For example, patients who cannot walk a block will also be unable to walk a mile and, hence, the second question would be redundant information. CAT works on a different principle, whereby a bank of validated items is used to develop a score for the construct (latent trait) that is being measured. The patient will be presented with an item of known difficulty and, based on the response to that question, additional items will be pulled from the bank to improve the precision of the estimate of that person's level of health or disability. The advantage of this approach is that within 6 or 7 questions, a firm estimate can usually be established. Although different patients will be answering different questions, it is still possible to establish a score because the level of difficulty of these items has been predetermined. This method is different from patient-specific PRO, in which the level of difficulty of the items that people self-select is not known. CAT has the potential to allow for concepts to be measured more expediently. The NIH has developed substantial efforts to develop such item banks and to validate them through the PROMIS network (http://www.nihpromis.org/measures/availableinstruments). This initiative has made substantial contributions to clinical measurement, including the development of clinical measurement methodologies and CAT item banks. The work is not complete, as many domains have not yet been fully validated. In fact, PROMIS also provides short forms of standardized items, recognizing that CAT does not meet all users' needs. One of the barriers to using CAT is that integrating technology into clinical practice or across multiple research sites can be challenging.

Where CAT is integrated into practice, it can help support the development of large databases of patient outcomes that can be used for secondary data analysis. Large-volume effectiveness research based on this type of data collection has the potential to help clinicians to better understand how interventions work in practice and which factors mediate patient outcomes.

REFERENCES

1. MacDermid JC. An introduction to evidence-based practice for hand therapists. J Hand Ther 2004;17: 105–17.

2. Szabo RM, MacDermid JC. An introduction to evidence-based practice for hand surgeons and therapists. Hand Clin 2009;25:1–14.

3. MacDermid JC, Grewal R, Macintyre NJ. Using an evidence-based approach to measure outcomes in clinical practice. Hand Clin 2009;25:97–111.

4. Sackett DL, Rosenberg WM, Gray JA, et al. Evidence based medicine: what it is and what it isn't. BMJ 1996;312:71–2.

5. Montori VM, Brito JP, Murad MH. The optimal practice of evidence-based medicine: incorporating patient preferences in practice guidelines. JAMA 2013;310:2503–4.

6. Richter B. Criteria for decision-making—what makes sense? Eur J Pediatr 2003;162(Suppl 1):S8–12.

7. Trevena L, Barratt A. Integrated decision making: definitions for a new discipline. Patient Educ Couns 2003;50:265–8.

8. Department of Health and Human Services, Food and Drug Administration Center for Drug Evaluation and Research, Center for Biologics Evaluation and Research, et al. Guidance for industry patient-reported outcome measures: use in medical product development to support labeling claims. Available at: http://www.fda.gov/downloads/Drugs/Guidances/UCM193282.pdf. 2009. Accessed February 02, 2014.

9. Abrams D, Davidson M, Harrick J, et al. Monitoring the change: current trends in outcome measure usage in physiotherapy. Man Ther 2006;11: 46–53.

10. Kay TM, Myers AM, Huijbregt MP. How far have we come since 1992? A comparative survey of physiotherapists' use of outcome measures. Physiother Can 2001;53:268–75.

11. MacDermid JC, Walton DM, Cote P, et al. Use of outcome measures in managing neck pain: an international multidisciplinary survey. Open Orthop J 2013;7:506–20.

12. Michlovitz SL, LaStayo PC, Alzner S, et al. Distal radius fractures: therapy practice patterns. J Hand Ther 2001;14:249–57.

13. MacDermid JC, Vincent JI, Kieffer L, et al. A survey of practice patterns for rehabilitation post elbow fracture. Open Orthop J 2012;6:429–39.

14. Cella DF. Quality of life: concepts and definition. J Pain Symptom Manage 1994;9:186–92.

15. Hayry M. Measuring the quality of life: why, how and what? Theor Med 1991;12:97–116.

16. Ventegodt S, Hilden J, Merrick J. Measurement of quality of life I. A methodological framework. ScientificWorldJournal 2003;3:950–61.

17. Beaton DE, Katz JN, Fossel AH, et al. Measuring the whole or the parts? Validity, reliability, and responsiveness of the Disabilities of the Arm, Shoulder and Hand outcome measure in different regions of the upper extremity. J Hand Ther 2001;14:128–46.

18. Solway S, Beaton DE, McConnell S, et al. The Dash Outcome Measure User's Manual. 2nd edition. Ontario (Canada): Institute for Health and Work; 2002.

19. MacDermid JC, Turgeon T, Richards RS, et al. Patient rating of wrist pain and disability: a reliable and valid measurement tool. J Orthop Trauma 1998;12:577–86.

20. MacDermid JC. The Patient-Rated Wrist Evaluation (PRWE)© user manual. Available at: http://www.srs-mcmaster.ca/Portals/20/pdf/research_resources/PRWE_PRWHEUserManual_Dec2007.pdf. 2007. Accessed February 02, 2014.

21. MacDermid JC. Development of a scale for patient rating of wrist pain and disability. J Hand Ther 1996;9:178–83.

22. Beaton DE, Richards RR. Measuring function of the shoulder. A cross-sectional comparison of five questionnaires. J Bone Joint Surg Am 1996;78:882–90.

23. Soldatis JJ, Moseley JB, Etminan M. Shoulder symptoms in healthy athletes: a comparison of outcome scoring systems. J Shoulder Elbow Surg 1997;6:265–71.

24. Levine DW, Simmons SP, Koris MJ, et al. A self-administered questionnaire for assessment of severity of symptoms and functional status in carpal tunnel syndrome. J Bone Joint Surg Am 1993;75:1585–92.

25. Melzack R. The McGill pain questionnaire: major properties and scoring methods. Pain 1975;1:277–99.

26. Melzack R. The short-form McGill Pain Questionnaire. Pain 1987;30:191–7.

27. Osman A, Barrios FX, Kopper BA, et al. Factor structure, reliability, and validity of the Pain Catastrophizing Scale. J Behav Med 1997;20:589–605.

28. Sullivan MJ, Stanish W, Waite H, et al. Catastrophizing, pain, and disability in patients with soft-tissue injuries. Pain 1998;77:253–60.

29. Gilworth G, Chamberlain MA, Harvey A, et al. Development of a work instability scale for rheumatoid arthritis. Arthritis Rheum 2003;49:349–54.

30. Tang K, Beaton DE, Lacaille D, et al. The Work Instability Scale for Rheumatoid Arthritis (RA-WIS): does it work in osteoarthritis? Qual Life Res 2010;19:1057–68.

31. Roy JS, MacDermid JC, Amick BC III, et al. Validity and responsiveness of presenteeism scales in chronic work-related upper-extremity disorders. Phys Ther 2011;91:254–66.

32. Arumugam V, MacDermid JC. The work instability scale. J Phys 2013;59:212.

33. Carswell A, McColl MA, Baptiste S, et al. The Canadian Occupational Performance Measure: a research and clinical literature review. Can J Occup Ther 2004;71:210–22.

34. Kjeken I, Slatkowsky-Christensen B, Kvien TK, et al. Norwegian version of the Canadian occupational performance measure in patients with hand osteoarthritis: validity, responsiveness, and feasibility. Arthritis Rheum 2004;51:709–15.

35. Law M, Polatajko H, Pollock N, et al. Pilot testing of the Canadian Occupational Performance Measure: clinical and measurement issues. Can J Occup Ther 1994;61:191–7.

36. Law M, Baptiste S, McColl M, et al. The Canadian occupational performance measure: an outcome measure for occupational therapy. Can J Occup Ther 1990;57:82–7.

37. Sterling M, Brentnall D. Patient specific functional scale. Aust J Physiother 2007;53:65.

38. McMillan CR, Binhammer PA. Which outcome measure is the best? Evaluating responsiveness of the disabilities of the arm, shoulder, and hand questionnaire, the Michigan Hand Questionnaire and the patient-specific functional scale following hand and wrist surgery. Hand (N Y) 2009;4(3):311–8.

39. Westaway MD, Stratford PW, Binkley JM. The patient-specific functional scale: validation of its use in persons with neck dysfunction. J Orthop Sports Phys Ther 1998;27:331–8.

40. Case-Smith J. Outcomes in hand rehabilitation using occupational therapy services. Am J Occup Ther 2003;57:499–506.

41. Kjeken I, Dagfinrud H, Slatkowsky-Christensen B, et al. Activity limitations and participation restrictions in women with hand osteoarthritis: patients descriptions, and associations between dimensions of functioning. Ann Rheum Dis 2005;64:1633–8.

42. Cook KF, Dunn W, Griffith JW, et al. Pain assessment using the NIH Toolbox. Neurology 2013;80:S49–53.

43. London DA, Stepan JG, Boyer MI, et al. Performance characteristics of the verbal QuickDASH. J Hand Surg Am 2014;39:100–7.

44. Downie WW, Leatham PA, Rhind VM. Studies with pain rating scales. Ann Rheum Dis 1978;37:378–81.

45. Jensen MP, Dworkin RH, Gammaitoni AR, et al. Do pain qualities and spatial characteristics make independent contributions to interference with physical and emotional functioning? J Pain 2006;7:644–53.

46. Melzack R. The McGill pain questionnaire: from description to measurement. Anesthesiology 2005;103:199–202.

47. Strand LI, Ljunggren AE, Bogen B, et al. The Short-Form McGill Pain Questionnaire as an outcome measure: test-retest reliability and responsiveness to change. Eur J Pain 2008;12:917–25.

48. Adelmanesh F, Jalali A, Attarian H, et al. Reliability, validity, and sensitivity measures of expanded and

revised version of the short-form McGill Pain Questionnaire (SF-MPQ-2) in Iranian patients with neuropathic and non-neuropathic pain. Pain Med 2012;13:1631–6.

49. Ferreira KA, de Andrade DC, Teixeira MJ. Development and validation of a Brazilian version of the short-form McGill pain questionnaire (SF-MPQ). Pain Manag Nurs 2013;14:210–9.

50. MacDermid JC, Tottenham V. Responsiveness of the disability of the arm, shoulder, and hand (DASH) and patient-rated wrist/hand evaluation (PRWHE) in evaluating change after hand therapy. J Hand Ther 2004;17:18–23.

51. MacDermid JC. Outcome evaluation in patients with elbow pathology: issues in instrument development and evaluation. J Hand Ther 2001;14: 105–14.

52. MacDermid J. Update: the patient-rated forearm evaluation questionnaire is now the patient-rated tennis elbow evaluation. J Hand Ther 2005;18: 407–10.

53. MacDermid JC, Grewal R. Development and validation of the patient-rated ulnar nerve evaluation. BMC Musculoskelet Disord 2013;14:146.

54. Osman A, Barrios FX, Gutierrez PM, et al. The Pain Catastrophizing Scale: further psychometric evaluation with adult samples. J Behav Med 2000;23: 351–65.

55. Bellamy N, Campbell J, Haraoui B, et al. Development of the Australian/Canadian (AUSCAN) osteoarthritis (OA) hand index. Arthritis Rheum 1997; 40:863–9.

56. Bellamy N, Campbell J, Haraoui B, et al. Clinimetric properties of the AUSCAN Osteoarthritis Hand Index: an evaluation of reliability, validity and responsiveness. Osteoarthr Cartil 2002;10:863–9.

57. Rompe JD, Overend TJ, MacDermid JC. Validation of the patient-rated tennis elbow evaluation questionnaire. J Hand Ther 2007;20:3–11.

58. Rouleau DM, Faber K, MacDermid JC. Systematic review of patient-administered shoulder functional scores on instability. J Shoulder Elbow Surg 2010; 19:1121–8.

59. Beaton DE, Wright JG, Katz JN. Development of the QuickDASH: comparison of three item-reduction approaches. J Bone Joint Surg Am 2005;87: 1038–46.

60. Stratford PW, Binkley JM, Stratford DM. Development and initial validation of upper extremity functional index. Physiother Can 2005;281(53): 259–67.

61. Hiller LB, Wade CK. Upper extremity functional assessment scales in children with Duchenne muscular dystrophy. Arch Phys Med Rehabil 1992;73:527–34.

62. Chung KC, Pillsbury MS, Walters MR, et al. Reliability and validity testing of the Michigan Hand Outcomes Questionnaire. J Hand Surg Am 1998; 23:575–87.

63. Chung KC, Hamill JB, Walters MR, et al. The Michigan Hand Outcomes Questionnaire (MHQ): assessment of responsiveness to clinical change. Ann Plast Surg 1999;42:619–22.

64. Kotsis SV, Chung KC. Responsiveness of the Michigan Hand Outcomes Questionnaire and the Disabilities of the Arm, Shoulder and Hand questionnaire in carpal tunnel surgery. J Hand Surg Am 2005;30:81–6.

65. King GJ, Richards RR, Zuckerman JD, et al. A standardized method for assessment of elbow function. Research Committee, American Shoulder and Elbow Surgeons. J Shoulder Elbow Surg 1999; 8:351–4.

66. Roach KE, Budiman-Mak E, Songsiridej N, et al. Development of a shoulder pain and disability index. Arthritis Care Res 1991;4:143–9.

67. Williams JW Jr, Holleman DR Jr, Simel DL. Measuring shoulder function with the shoulder pain and disability index. J Rheumatol 1995;22:727–32.

68. Roy JS, MacDermid JC, Faber KJ, et al. The simple shoulder test is responsive in assessing change following shoulder arthroplasty. J Orthop Sports Phys Ther 2010;40:413–21.

69. Matsen FA III, Ziegler DW, DeBartolo SE. Patient self-assessment of health status and function in glenohumeral degenerative joint disease. J Shoulder Elbow Surg 1995;4:345–51.

70. Lerner D, Amick BC III, Rogers WH, et al. The work limitations questionnaire. Med Care 2001; 39:72–85.

71. Lerner D, Reed JI, Massarotti E, et al. The Work Limitations Questionnaire's validity and reliability among patients with osteoarthritis. J Clin Epidemiol 2002;55:197–208.

72. Hughes RE, Johnson ME, Skow A, et al. Reliability of a simple shoulder endurance test. J Musculoskelet Res 1999;3:195–200.

73. Tang K, Beaton DE, Boonen A, et al. Measures of work disability and productivity: Rheumatoid Arthritis Specific Work Productivity Survey (WPS-RA), Workplace Activity Limitations Scale (WALS), Work Instability Scale for Rheumatoid Arthritis (RA-WIS), Work Limitations Questionnaire (WLQ), and Work Productivity and Activity Impairment Questionnaire (WPAI). Arthritis Care Res (Hoboken) 2011;63(Suppl 11):S337–49.

74. Topolski TD, LoGerfo J, Patrick DL, et al. The Rapid Assessment of Physical Activity (RAPA) among older adults. Prev Chronic Dis 2006;3:A118.

75. University of Washington Health Promotion Research Center. RAPA - rapid assessment of physical activity. Seattle (WA): University of Washington, Health Promotion Research Center; 2006. Available at: http://depts.washington.edu/hprc/rapa.

76. Alvarez C, Kirkley A, Griffin S, et al. The development and evaluation of a disease specific quality of life measurement tool for rotator cuff disease. Clin J Sport Med 1998;26(6):764–72.

77. Lo IK, Griffin S, Kirkley A. The development of a disease-specific quality of life measurement tool for osteoarthritis of the shoulder: the Western Ontario Osteoarthritis of the Shoulder (WOOS) index. Osteoarthr Cartil 2001;9:771–8.

78. Colquhoun HL, Letts LJ, Law MC, et al. Administration of the Canadian Occupational Performance Measure: effect on practice. Can J Occup Ther 2012;79:120–8.

79. MacDermid JC, Walton DM, Miller J, et al. What is the experience of receiving healthcare for neck pain? Open Orthop J 2013;7:428–39.

80. MacDermid JC, Roth JH, McMurtry R. Predictors of time lost from work following a distal radius fracture. J Occup Rehabil 2007;17:47–62.

81. Novak CB, Anastakis DJ, Beaton DE, et al. Biomedical and psychosocial factors associated with disability after peripheral nerve injury. J Bone Joint Surg Am 2011;93:929–36.

82. Vranceanu AM, Bachoura A, Weening A, et al. Psychological factors predict disability and pain intensity after skeletal trauma. J Bone Joint Surg Am 2014;96:e20.

83. Wertli MM, Eugster R, Held U, et al. Catastrophizing—a prognostic factor for outcome in patients with low back pain - a systematic review. Spine J 2014. [Epub ahead of print].

84. Jahagirdar D, Kroll T, Ritchie K, et al. Using patient reported outcome measures in health services: a qualitative study on including people with low literacy skills and learning disabilities. BMC Health Serv Res 2012;12:431.

85. Adams J, Chapman J, Bradley S, et al. Literacy levels required to complete routinely used patient-reported outcome measures in rheumatology. Rheumatology (Oxford) 2013;52:460–4.

86. Willis DB. Cognitive interviewing: a "how to" guide. Available at: http://appliedresearch.cancer.gov/areas/cognitive/interview.pdf. 1999. Accessed February 02, 2014.

87. Cibelli K. Cognitive interviewing techniques: a brief overview. Available at: http://www.metagora.org/training/example/SL_1_CognitiveInterviewing_051405.pdf. 1994. Accessed February 02, 2014.

88. Farrar JT, Pritchett YL, Robinson M, et al. The clinical importance of changes in the 0 to 10 numeric rating scale for worst, least, and average pain intensity: analyses of data from clinical trials of duloxetine in pain disorders. J Pain 2010;11:109–18.

89. Tennant A, McKenna SP, Hagell P. Application of Rasch analysis in the development and application of quality of life instruments. Value Health 2004;7(Suppl 1):S22–6.

90. Tennant A, Conaghan PG. The Rasch measurement model in rheumatology: what is it and why use it? When should it be applied, and what should one look for in a Rasch paper? Arthritis Rheum 2007;57:1358–62.

91. Cieza A, Brockow T, Ewert T, et al. Linking health-status measurements to the international classification of functioning, disability and health. J Rehabil Med 2002;34:205–10.

92. Lohmann S, Decker J, Muller M, et al. The ICF forms a useful framework for classifying individual patient goals in post-acute rehabilitation. J Rehabil Med 2011;43:151–5.

93. Stucki G, Cieza A, Ewert T, et al. Application of the International Classification of Functioning, Disability and Health (ICF) in clinical practice. Disabil Rehabil 2002;24:281–2.

94. Stucki G, Ewert T, Cieza A. Value and application of the ICF in rehabilitation medicine. Disabil Rehabil 2002;24:932–8.

95. Schwarzkopf SR, Ewert T, Dreinhofer KE, et al. Towards an ICF Core Set for chronic musculoskeletal conditions: commonalities across ICF Core Sets for osteoarthritis, rheumatoid arthritis, osteoporosis, low back pain and chronic widespread pain. Clin Rheumatol 2008;27:1355–61.

96. Cieza A, Ewert T, Ustun TB, et al. Development of ICF Core Sets for patients with chronic conditions. J Rehabil Med 2004;(Suppl 44):9–11.

97. Dreinhofer K, Stucki G, Ewert T, et al. ICF Core Sets for osteoarthritis. J Rehabil Med 2004;134(Suppl 44):75–80.

98. Goldhahn J, Beaton D, Ladd A, et al. Recommendation for measuring clinical outcome in distal radius fractures: a core set of domains for standardized reporting in clinical practice and research. Arch Orthop Trauma Surg 2014;134:197–205.

Bench to Bedside
Integrating Advances in Basic Science into Daily Clinical Practice

Rory B. McGoldrick, MD, FRCS(Plast), MBA*, Kenneth Hui, BA,
James Chang, MD

KEYWORDS

- Commercialization • Technology transfer process • Patenting • Marketing • Licensing
- Company startup • Food and Drugs Administration • Clinical trials

KEY POINTS

- Reconstructive surgery is evolving; there are significant clinical needs for which tissue engineering may provide an elegant solution.
- Negotiating the interface between scientific research and commercialization is often confounding.
- Working with a technology transfer office (TTO) will facilitate the commercialization process.
- Patent attorneys and TTO collaboration is encouraged.
- Patents may take up to 3 years to be granted.
- Marketing and licensing should be approached cautiously so that the best licensing deal is achieved.
- Startup company development is a high-risk proposition.
- Exclusive licensing deals are the gold standard for startups.
- TTOs will insist on all conflicts of interest being addressed if the inventor is affiliated with a university.
- Entrepreneurial advice is critical and business planning pivotal to the investment potential of startups.
- One should take advantage of the overabundance of informal routes of communication possible with the Food and Drug Administration to obtain timely and accurate feedback from the agency regarding specific products to ensure efficient progression of new products toward clinical trials in the United States.
- All current good manufacturing practice guidelines must be adhered to and will be routinely inspected.

INTRODUCTION

Everybody always wants to know what's next. I always say that what I can imagine is rather dull. What I can't imagine is what excites me.
—Arthur Schawlow, Stanford physicist and Nobel Laureate.

Hand and upper extremity surgeons still face reconstructive tissue shortages following trauma, tumor ablation, or congenital absence. This shortage is compounded by the innate anatomic intricacy within the hand that is crucial for its form and function.

Current needs are such that hand surgeons should be familiar with autologous free tissue

Disclosures: None of the authors have a relationship with commercial companies with conflicting financial interests within this article.
CME/CE Credits: None.
Section of Plastic Surgery, Division of Plastic and Reconstructive Surgery, Stanford University Medical Center, VA Palo Alto Health Care System, 770 Welch Road, Suite 400, Palo Alto, CA 94304, USA
* Corresponding author.
E-mail address: rorymcg@stanford.edu

Hand Clin 30 (2014) 305–317
http://dx.doi.org/10.1016/j.hcl.2014.04.004
0749-0712/14/$ – see front matter Published by Elsevier Inc.

hand.theclinics.com

transfer and the immunologic and technical aspects of composite tissue allotransplantation. Indeed, vascularized composite allotransplantation has become increasingly practiced internationally following developments in microsurgical techniques, organ transplantation, and immunosuppression.[1] The technique, however, is still plagued by poor immune-tolerance profiles and the significant morbidity associated with pharmacologic immunosuppression.[1–3]

Therefore, in recent years great interest has developed in tissue engineering (TE) and regenerative medicine in reconstructive hand surgery. This concept combines the principles of life sciences and engineering in developing biological substitutes that will restore, maintain, or improve hand-tissue function. These frontiers are currently the focus of intense international surgical innovation efforts as a means of recapturing the natural form and function of the hand.

In addition to other surgical discoveries, TE is the catalyst for advances in clinical care, particularly in hand surgery, whereby many unmet clinical needs remain and useful inventions in this area could considerably improve the lives of patients. The challenge remains for the surgeon-scientist to successfully negotiate the path from new technology to the bedside of patients.

The process of discovery, invention, and subsequent commercialization of a product often takes substantial investment of time and money, and involves a substantial financial risk. Such investment can prove too much for most medical device start-ups, 90% of which do not progress to clinical trials.[4]

Many hand surgeons have new ideas with real commercial potential, but are not equipped with the tools to take such ideas forward. Plastic surgery is a specialty dependent on a rich heritage of innovation, so it is paramount that clinicians become enlightened in the process of taking ideas from the bench to the bedside.

This article focuses on the initial steps of commercial development of a patentable scientific discovery through to the marketing of a clinical product. First, the basic strategy of partnering with a technology transfer office (TTO) and the complex process of patenting are addressed. Next, marketing and licensing the patent to a company, in addition to starting a company, is discussed. Finally, the basics of obtaining clearance from the Food and Drugs Administration (FDA), production in a good manufacturing practice (GMP) facility, and bringing the product to clinical trial are addressed.

PARTNERING WITH A TECHNOLOGY TRANSFER OFFICE

The First Critical Steps After a Scientific Discovery

Antecedent to the pursuit of any funding streams, the time period following the discovery of a surgical innovation may be arguably the most critical to the idea successfully reaching patients. Intellectual property (IP) law is the legal field that establishes, protects, and arbitrates the ownership of the inventor's original ideas. The IP strategy for a university affiliated surgeon-scientist should start as soon as a discovery is made.

If one feels a discovery is worthy of patent protection, it is critical to avoid publicly disclosing this idea, as one may risk forfeiting rights to the IP. One should avoid publication, and even presentation at local meetings. It is essential to meticulously document the development of one's idea in the event that originality is contested. The process should be recorded in ink, with the use of pictures as appropriate, in a secure laboratory notebook, with countersignatures of a lay person for verification purposes.

In the United States, the inventor may have only 1 year to file a patent application to protect the IP from the time of initial public disclosure or effort at commercialization. If the inventor filed for a foreign patent more than 1 year before the domestic application, the domestic application will be disqualified. A 1-year period of grace does not exist for most foreign patents, so to capture foreign markets it is important to file the patent application before any public disclosure.[5]

The Role of the TTO and the Technology Transfer Process

A reliable framework for commercializing discoveries for the aspiring surgeon entrepreneur should include working with a TTO or an office that performs a similar function, which will protect an institution's IP and propel research efforts to commercialization by turning scientific progress into tangible products, while returning income to both the inventor and the university to support further research, as outlined in **Fig. 1**.

This competitive process starts with the submission of an Invention Disclosure. This written notice of invention begins the formal technology transfer process. It is a confidential document, and should fully describe the new aspects of the invention, including the critical solution it provides and its advantages and benefits over current technologies.

The office will work with the inventor to make an initial assessment concerning patentability,

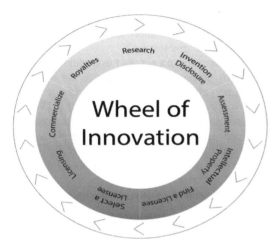

Fig. 1. The wheel of innovation of a typical technology transfer office.

technical feasibility, and commercial potential of the invention, and make a preliminary judgment about the potential to create a startup company.

If the application is promising, the TTO will assign the disclosure to a licensing associate who will formally review the discovery and evaluate the discovery's commercialization potential based on patent searches, market analysis, and existing competitive technologies. This assessment will ultimately guide the licensing strategy.

The first step in this process is a comprehensive patent and literature search to confirm that the idea is indeed novel before any patent is applied for. This question is usually answered through an initial search of the United States Patent and Trademark Office (USPTO) (http://www.uspto.gov/patft/index.html) or the World Intellectual Property Organization (www.wipo.int) databases. One can also search the full text of all United States patents via the Google Patent Search function.

The prior art search should be conducted with the assistance of a patent attorney. Prior art is any body of knowledge that relates to the invention, including previous patents, journal articles, other publications, meeting presentations or abstracts, trade shows, or public use or sales anywhere in the world. This search maximizes all potential applications covered in the patent in addition to conceiving a myriad of applications not envisaged by the inventor, and will protect not only the idea but also the multitude of approaches by which competitors could circumvent IP protection.

Assuming that the disclosure passes these hurdles and the TTO feels that the scientific discovery is likely be a new hand surgery entity, novel and patentable, a strategy is drafted to seek protection and coverage for the relevant clinical uses. A patent counsel drafts a patent application; depending on the nature of the discovery and strength of the supporting data, either a provisional or a regular application may be filed with the USPTO and/or foreign agencies as required.

A best-practice IP strategy is to brainstorm in conjunction with a surgical innovation team, preferably with members having commercial experience in biotechnology, and a patent counsel highly knowledgable in the field relating to the discovery. The goal is to build a road map for disclosing and filing applications that will enable any potential startup to establish a solid ring around the technology platform and its potential use, deter any competition, extend the time frame of patent protection, and, obviously, build a source of revenue from out-licensing activities. This process will be iterative and evolve over time as a startup continues to build and grow from a preclinical to the clinical development stage.

THE INTRICACIES OF PATENTING A SCIENTIFIC DISCOVERY
Definition and Purpose

A patent is a document granted by the US Government that provides a form of limited monopoly. It is not a guarantee of rights or, indeed, an exclusive right to practice the invention defined in the patent. It is designed only with the right to stop others using the IP. It grants the holder the right to stop others from making, using, selling, or distributing the patented invention for the lifetime of the patent. The patent holder has the right to file a lawsuit against the accused infringer of the patent for financial damages, in addition to an injunction.

Patent protection begins with the filing of a patent application with the USPTO and, when appropriate, foreign patent offices. Once a patent application has been filed, it requires several years and tens of thousands of dollars to obtain an issued patent. As a consequence of advancing technology and growing awareness of the value of patents, the past 20 years has seen an explosion in the number of patent applications with year-on-year increases. In 2012, the USPTO took in 542,815 utility patent applications and granted 276,788 of these.[5]

The issuance of a patent is not inevitable. Indeed, in the United States and most of the world a patent will not be granted, even if you are the inventor, if the invention was disclosed publicly first, if someone else filed a patent application on the invention first, or there was a failure to provide enough information in the patent application so that someone could understand and practice the invention. There are certain exceptions to these general concepts; the reader is therefore advised to seek advice from a patent attorney or patent agent as soon as a discovery is made, and certainly before any public disclosures.

International Patents

There are no truly worldwide patents, and a patent from the United States does not give the inventor any rights in other countries. Instead each country or region grants its own geographically limited monopoly. It must be remembered that one must initially file a patent application in one's home country to establish its presence for the rest of the world, and treaties such as the Paris Treaty (PT) and the Patent Cooperative Treaty (PCT) make this possible. Inventors in all countries can file their patent application in their home country, and know that as long as they file their international applications within 1 year from the day they filed their first application, they can derive benefit internationally as if they had filed it on that earlier date.

TTO and Patent Filing

The 1980 Bayh-Dole Act allowed and encouraged universities to own and commercialize patents resulting from the work of their associated researchers. Therefore, the integration of basic surgical science into clinical practice is facilitated by a strong relationship between the surgeon-scientist and the university's TTO.[6,7]

Only the original inventors may apply for the patent, and if the inventor works for a corporation or university there is an obligation to sign one's scientific discovery to that institution, after which the patent will be issued to the inventor and assigned to the institution.

Leahy-Smith America Invents Act

In the United States, traditionally the patent was awarded to the first person to invent the product, not the first person to file the patent on the invention. By meticulous laboratory documentation the inventor proved that he or she was the person with the original idea.

President Obama signed into law the Leahy-Smith America Invents Act (AIA) on September 16, 2011 which, on March 16, 2013, changed the law from a "first to invent" to a "first to file" system. This change brought the process in line with most patent jurisdictions worldwide. Thus, if 2 individuals separately apply for patents on the same invention, the patent will go to the inventor who filed a patent application first, regardless of any laboratory documentation (assuming there was no prior public disclosure).[8]

This new ruling preserves the traditional 1-year period of grace for an inventor to file a patent application after making a public disclosure. However, the inventor must check with the TTO, or equivalent, for specific policies. For example, the Stanford University Office of Technology and Licensing has made the decision that it will not file a patent application if the invention has been publicly disclosed before filing, as it considers it makes more sense strategically to proceed as if the United States had transitioned to a true "first to file" system, such as that in Europe.[9]

Provisional Patent Application

If the inventor wishes to protect the IP but chooses to delay some of the expense necessary to apply for a formal patent application, he or she can file for a provisional patent application. Associated costs are much lower than that of a formal patent, and the application is not published or examined. This approach provides patent protection for 1 year, but one has to apply for a formal utility patent application within that year.

During this year, if the IP is disclosed and the inventor chooses to abandon the original patent application, he or she cannot seek patent protection for the scientific discovery. This approach is best suited to individuals who wish to delay the application, allowing time to ensure the idea is worthwhile.[10]

Patent Types

The USPTO recognizes 3 types of patents. A utility patent, the most common type, refers to inventions that have a particular function. By contrast, design patents cover nonfunctional parts of articles, such as the unique, ornamental shape or surface of an item. Lastly, a plant patent protects inventions of asexually reproducible plants.

Utility patents cover new articles of manufacture, processes, or machines, and are issued for a term of 20 years from the date of the application.[11] These patents are the most relevant to the hand surgeon, and are therefore the focus of the following discussion. For the scientific discovery to be regarded as a utility it must have a useful purpose beyond knowledge, and must be able to be used to do something, make something, or treat something.[12]

Patent Requirements

A patent can be rejected for many reasons, such as failing the novelty and nonobviousness requirements. Novelty means it is different from the prior art (previous patents or something known to the public). The disclosure must be public and can take many forms but, for purposes of patent law, public means it could be seen or could be found, not actually seen or found. The invention must be nonobvious to someone who is skilled in the art (knowledgable in the field of interest). Nonobviousness means that the invention is different enough from prior art that someone skilled in the area of technology would not consider the idea obvious.

Steps in Obtaining a Patent

Surgeon-scientists may navigate the process on their own under the auspices of being pro se (representing oneself), but again it is recommended that counsel from expert patent attorneys and the TTO, if available, is sought. Indeed, once the primary application is submitted it is essential for an attorney to navigate the inventor through the prosecution process.

An application can be submitted electronically through the USPTO Web site, by mail, or by fax. Applications can be a utility patent (a full and complete application that has the possibility of becoming a patent) or a provisional application, a foreign patent application, or a PCT application. Specifications for the formal utility patent application are shown in **Table 1**.

Table 1
Specifications of a typical utility patent application

Section	Description
Abstract	A summary of the rest of the specification
Background	Describes the need for your invention and problems that your invention solves
Summary	Short explanation of the invention
Detailed description	Includes a description of the ideal embodiment, as well as additional embodiments of the invention and how it works
Conclusion, ramification, and scope	Briefly states the advantages of the invention and the additional embodiments again, as well as how the legal scope should not be limited to forms shown

The time course for the process depends on the kind of application and the technology involved; it can take 1 to 3 years before a patent is granted, as shown in **Fig. 2**.

The inventor will work with one patent examiner throughout the process, and the process of give and take between the inventor and the USPTO is called prosecution. It is very rare for an examiner to grant an allowance to a patent on the first attempt. More than likely, the examiner will give a nonfinal rejection that allows amendment of claims, elaboration, or both. The overall process for obtaining a patent is outlined in **Fig. 3**.

MARKETING AND LICENSING THE PATENT TO A COMPANY
Going Solo

Once the IP of the discovery has been secured, surgeon-scientists who do not wish to start a company have to license their invention. Licensing allows a company to commercialize whatever aspect of the IP is licensed, and as consideration for this right the inventor will receive royalties.

If one company licenses exclusive rights of the patent in all fields, it has unrestricted use of all the applications of the patented IP. A field of use license may be issued to license specific applications to different companies. Patent holders may issue exclusive or nonexclusive licenses. The downside is that one has less control over the process and potentially less profit from the patent. However, this should not understate the benefit from not having to negotiate the FDA approval process, and the manufacture, marketing, and sale of the product.

Although many surgeons would prefer to let the TTO handle the licensing, this is not always an option if the discovery has not been accepted for technology transfer by the office. If this is the case, the first step is to find companies that may be interested in the patent or, indeed, any derived products. Companies that manufacture products similar to the discovery in question would be ideal, but would benefit from adding the patent to their repertoire. Alternatively, new ventures may be sought from companies with no experience in these areas.

The key to the next stage is winning the business by demonstrating a solid proof of concept and niche-market landscape. During these stages it is recommended that an attorney be present to guide one through the process and also in drafting a license agreement.

Marketing and Licensing with a TTO

The TTO will broadly market the technology to appropriate companies that could be interested

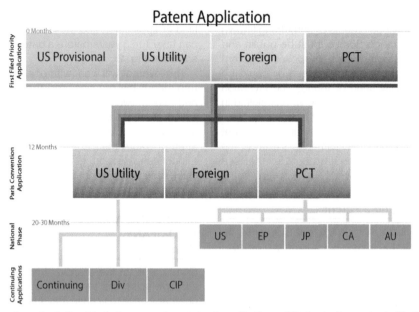

Fig. 2. Time scale and relationship between various patent applications. AU, Australian patent; CA, Canadian patent; CIP, continuation in part; Div, divisional; EP, European patent; JP, Japanese patent; PCT, Patent Cooperative Treaty.

in commercializing a particular invention. With the inventor's input, the TTO creates a marketing overview of the technology and identifies candidate licensing companies that have the expertise, resources, and business networks to bring the technology to market and, thus, to the patient's bedside.

Of crucial importance is that inventors are discouraged from directly being involved in the TTO licensing process negotiations with potential licensees (including startup scenarios), owing to conflicts of interest from potential roles including surgeon researcher, royalty recipient, company consultant, and company board member.

The TTOs will broadly market most technologies, including those with startup interest for up to 6 months before the licensing associate selects a licensee. This action helps mitigate and manage conflicts of interest if the surgeon-scientist is considering licensing for a startup company. Moreover, under the Bayh-Dole Act a University has an implicit obligation to ensure that inventions funded by the federal government are effectively commercialized.

Once a party has been identified as a suitable licensee, the TTO will normally negotiate and execute a license or option agreement. This document is a contract between the university or corporation and a company, in which certain rights to a surgical technology are granted to a company in return for financial and other benefits. In some instances, if the surgeon-scientist wishes to have a managerial role in a startup company he or she may have to forgo their university affiliations, and individuals are advised to seek TTO advice on this matter.

TTO Licensing for Startup Companies

Many individuals who wish to form a startup company request an exclusive license which, it is believed, allows for the optimum fundraising for that company. In this situation, licensing to that company will obviously raise concerns about conflicts of commitment and interest. Most TTOs cannot sign off any agreements until the appropriate conflict of interest reviews and approvals are completed.

Exclusive licensees are generally expected to pay patent expenses, and other financial terms may also include a small, minority share of equity in the company. The TTO will be likely to also enforce field-of-use restrictions because a startup company often does not have the resources to develop all the applications of an invention, and diligence terms to ensure reasonable progress in growing the company and commercializing the invention.

STARTING A COMPANY

Formation of a new company is a high-risk proposition, and the inventor-entrepreneur should be cautious when starting a new company, as there are many potential pitfalls. Although most TTOs

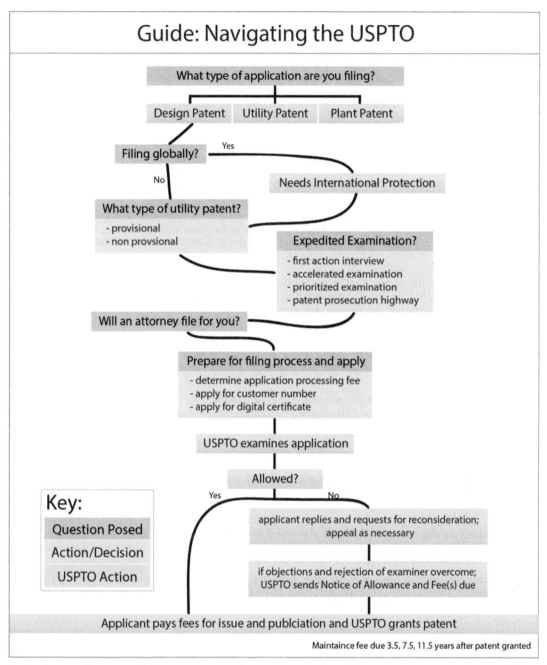

Guide: Navigating the USPTO

What type of application are you filing?

Design Patent   Utility Patent   Plant Patent

Filing globally?   Yes

No

Needs International Protection

What type of utility patent?
- provisional
- non provsional

Expedited Examination?
- first action interview
- accelerated examination
- prioritized examination
- patent prosecution highway

Will an attorney file for you?

Prepare for filing process and apply
- determine application processing fee
- apply for customer number
- apply for digital certificate

USPTO examines application

Allowed?
Yes   No

applicant replies and requests for reconsideration; appeal as necessary

if objections and rejection of examiner overcome; USPTO sends Notice of Allowance and Fee(s) due

Key:
Question Posed
Action/Decision
USPTO Action

Applicant pays fees for issue and publciation and USPTO grants patent

Maintaince fee due 3.5, 7.5, 11.5 years after patent granted

Fig. 3. The overall process of filing a patent application. USPTO, United States Patent and Trademark Office.

will play a relatively passive role in company formation, some may actively engage in writing a business plan, assist in the formation of the company, sourcing seed funding, recruiting a management team, and securing a first round of venture funding.[13] Thus it is critical to work closely with the TTO.

Companies fail even when the core technology is innovative and promising. **Box 1** outlines several

pitfalls a startup company may face, with cautionary advice.

The Business Plan

Every startup business follows its own unique path and corporate structure (US Small Business Administration [www.sba.gov]). The most common startup company structure is that of a limited

---

Box 1
Common problems faced by startup companies

Patent problems

- One should avoid negotiating poor patent license terms that can retard the commercialization process or deter investors. The hand surgeon who intends to form a startup should ideally seek an exclusive license, preferably exclusive for the life of the patent period, in conjunction with terms that are favorable to attract investors.

Licensing issues

- The licensing agreement should contain, at a minimum, the length of the exclusivity, field of use, any improvement on the invention, assignment provisions, and financial terms. A license should have as few limitations as possible. The ability to assign licensing rights is important so as not to impede potential investment and exit opportunities for the spinout.

- The TTOs will charge license fees, which may represent a significant impediment for an aspiring surgical entrepreneur. In this case, the startup should prefer to trade equity for cash, ideally kept to a minimum with equity ownership, typically low (single digit), and subject to dilution as a substitute.

Financial constraints

- The royalty rate should be targeted at an industry norm. In some circumstances, the startup must also license from others to have the rights needed to create a licensed product, and should be prepared to negotiate for a reduction in the royalty rate. The TTO will require reimbursement for patent costs, but payments should be delayed until certain funding levels are reached.

- The licensing agreement may contain diligence terms (reaching specified funding level, reaching certain sales volume by a specific time frame), which can be very rigid while intending to ensure that the spinout does not lose its viability, and subsequently can lead to a loss on the university's initial investment.

- A startup needs sufficient capital to overcome technical challenges, reach critical business milestones, and progress to the next phase of development. To attract investors, the company must have a solid business plan and a strong management team.

Corporate concerns

- A strong connection between founders, management, and investors is required to buy into the same strategic vision. If there is a lack of startup or general business experience, or simply a breakdown in communication, problems may arise.

Market and Niche Logistics

- On occasion, despite a very innovative and exciting discovery, there is no market. Even when commercial needs exist the company may miss the market, as it is not ready, may be mistimed or too expensive, or have been replaced by competition at the last minute.

- If the target market has been overestimated (and the product has a marginal niche) through inaccurate research, the startup will simply not meet its financial targets.

---

liability company (LLC). This hybrid business entity has certain characteristics of both a corporation (because of the limited liability) and a partnership (because of pass through income taxation), or sole proprietorship.

If affiliated with a university, the support required in starting a business is commonly readily available in the form of entrepreneurship networks. In the early days, it is very important to network and to gain as much advice as possible before writing a business case, a typical framework of which is shown in **Box 2**.

A key question should concern how far along the technology is developed and how much further research is required; this must also include financial implications. This development risk is a key consideration for any potential investor. An investor will insist on a favorable development cost versus investment return.

One must be aware of the overall market into which the invention will be placed. Is the market large enough for a new technology and is there a healthy grown trend in the particular niche? Indeed, what market share will be obtained and is this financially viable? If not, one may consider different product strategies to allow the new technology to broaden into multiple product platforms to increase profit. This move is essential, as

---

Box 2
Typical composition of a startup business plan

A compelling proof of concept placed in the hand surgical context with a mission statement

Competitive advantage profile, to include IP protection strategy and current patent landscape (USPTO search results)

Market status with a projection of the invention's impact on the marketplace

Marketing and sales strategy with pricing, product, and placement plans

Financial potential of the invention

    Primary funding requirements (including that required to finish any further research)

    Financial projections over 5 to 10 years, to include when the startup breaks even and details of any equity share from TTO (detailing diligence terms)

    Key milestones (with metrics) required to meet the financial projections and key assumptions, and how these may change based on marketplace dynamics and competition

Proven management team and corporate structure

Timeline with key milestones of overall startup development stage

Overall risk factor and mitigation measures with an SWOT analysis: Strengths, Weaknesses, Opportunities, and Threats

---

investors demand startups with high growth potential.

Funding Revenues

Funding is required to initiate the commercialization of any invention. Investment capital for seed and early-stage investment is often a major hurdle in the ability of a university spinoff or startup to successfully commercialize discoveries. The aspiring surgeon-scientist entrepreneurs will find that commercializing their own discoveries with startup funds can be an enormous challenge. Several types of funding are available to obtain the required capital.

In the $5 to $10 million range, venture capital groups are the typical sources of startup funds. One may seek venture capital as a significant source of funding, but recent trends have shown venture capitalists fundamentally shifting to financing later-stage biotechnology and medical device companies only.[13–16] A venture capitalist will invest large sums of money in exchange for receiving an equity share. Venture capitalists tend to exercise significant control, and bring experienced management talent to help guide and grow the company.

Because this is a competitive source of funding, a solid business plan will need to be in place to compete for these resources.[17] Venture capital groups must be able to pay out to investors in 3 to 7 years; thus they will have an exit strategy that may or may not be favorable to the inventors. To secure the cash, the inventor should be prepared to potentially yield some control of the invention's development.[18–20]

Typically the venture capital group acquires a percentage ownership of the young company (often a controlling interest) and the ability to appoint some of the key managers within the corporate structure.[18] In general, the degree of control the venture capital group demands will correlate with its financial investment.

The recent downturn in early venture capital investment creates a significant challenge for individuals seeking investment in discovery and pre-clinical development programs.[21] Indeed, in the early stages many individuals raise funds on their own and through friends and family. However, a plethora of other funding streams have been explored to bridge any gaps in the early stages of a startup. These sources may be nondilutive and dilutive.

There are several grants from federal, regional, and state-based programs. Federal options include the Small Business Innovation Research (SBIR) (http://www.sba.gov/content/small-business-innovation-research-program-sbir) and Small Business Technology Transfer Research (SBTTR) (http://www.sba.gov/content/small-business-technology-transfer-program-sttr) grants. The goal of these grants is to foster commercialization of innovation derived from federally funded research and development.

These grants are advantageous because the inventions developed as a result of the grant are the property of the inventors and, as such, are not liable for payment of royalties to the government.

Obtaining this grant may move the technology further downstream before engaging private funders, a validation technical approach by subject matter experts, and access to sole-source status for some federal contracts associated with subsequent development of the technology. Qualification as a sole-source contractor can make a small business highly attractive to a larger public company for competitive advantage as a partner in large federal contracts.[22]

The SBTTR grant requires university partnering with the business, and the SBIR grant permits but does not require a university affiliation, so there is a degree of flexibility. The downside is that there are certain specific conditions, and obtaining the grant may take considerable time. If the inventor's patent has been filed, time may be critical.

Other nondilutive, nontraditional funding streams include banks, which do not typically participate in equity investments in startups but are obviously a source of loans, particularly for capital purchases when there is a degree of collateral. Finally, crowd funding can be used, whereby various companies enable entrepreneurial fund raising by pooling small investments from a network of individuals.

Angel investors are emerging as a significant source of funding for early-stage entrepreneurial ventures. The amount of investment capital from angel investing is substantial. According to the Q1Q2 2013 Angel Market Analysis Report by the Center for Venture Research at the University of New Hampshire, angel investments totaled $9.7 billion, an increase of 5.2% over Q1Q2 in 2012. Software accounted for the largest share of investments, with 24% of total angel investments in Q1Q2 in 2013, followed by Healthcare Services/Medical Devices and Equipment (21%).[23]

OBTAINING FDA CLEARANCE

The prerequisite for commercializing any discovery is to adequately address the regulatory requirements for demonstrating efficacy and safety, which is primarily dealt with by the FDA (www.fda.gov) and the Advanced Medical Technology Association, which sets out a code of ethics (http://advamed.org/issues/1/code-of-ethics).

A new scientific product is either a discrete entity covered by the innovator's patent or products that can be derived from the innovator's patent. The FDA classifies medical products into 3 main categories. A drug is a product that has an active ingredient that reacts or otherwise affects the person. A medical device is a product that is prosthetic or decellularized and may be implanted on or inside a person. Finally, a biological

product is regarded as any product with live cells within it.

As TE and regenerative medicine evolves, so do several combination products that fall between the categories of biomaterials and cell-based technologies. The FDA regards these as tissue-engineered medical products (TEMPs) that do not fit the 3 broad main categories. Most surgeon-scientist related products would fall into the category of medical devices or TEMPs.

Medical Devices

The FDA describes medical devices to include "medical implants" that consist of "devices or tissues that are placed inside or on the surface of the body." Indeed, "many implants are prosthetic, intended to replace missing body parts" and "other implants deliver medication, monitor body functions, or provide support to organs and tissues."[24]

This category would therefore include skin graft products and bone scaffolds, whose development and production is overseen by the Center for Devices and Radiological Health (CDRH). The CDRH, under the guidance of the Medical Devices Amendment of the Federal Food, Drug and Cosmetic Act of 1976, further classifies devices into 1 of 3 categories: Class I, Class II, or Class III.

These classifications are based on the level of regulation required to ensure safety and efficacy of the device. Examples of Class I devices include elastic bandages, examination gloves, and hand-held surgical instruments. Class II devices include infusion pumps and surgical drapes. Class III devices include heart valves, breast implants, and implanted cerebellar stimulators.

Once classified, the medical device will then be assigned to 1 of 3 approval pathways that guide its transition from prototype to market approval: exemption, 510(k) premarket notification, and premarket approval (PMA). All Class I/II devices undergo 510(k) premarket notification and Class III devices undergo the process of PMA. These rules apply unless a device exemption is in place.

Class I devices require the least strict regulation but are subject to general controls including establishment registration, medical device listing, device production in accordance with good manufacturing processes, and proper compliance with described labeling regulations.[25] Class II devices require further regulation to include special labeling requirements, performance standards, and postmarket surveillance.[25] Finally, most regulation falls on the Class III medical devices, whose approval poses the greatest risk. The FDA defines Class III devices as "those that support or sustain human life, are of substantial importance in preventing impairment of human health, or which present a potential, unreasonable risk of illness or injury."[26] All medical implants would be regarded as a Class III medical device.

Class I/II devices that are not exempt, in addition to Class III devices exempt from PMA, intended for use in humans are subject to the process of 510(k) premarket notification.[27] This process acts to establish that a medical device has substantial equivalence (SE) to 1 or more legally marketed devices (predicates). Ninety days following the submission of the 510(k), if successful, a notification declaring the device to have SE is issued, and marketing of the device may start. If an SE is not found then the medical device is regarded as Class III and undergoes further scrutiny in the form of a PMA.[28]

The PMA is a rigorous and detailed scientific and regulatory review to evaluate the safety and effectiveness of the Class II medical devices. FDA regulations provide 180 days to review the PMA and make a decision. The review time is normally very much longer in reality, and before approving or denying a PMA; the appropriate FDA advisory committee may review the PMA at a public meeting. After the FDA notifies the applicant that the PMA has been approved or denied, a notice is published on the Internet (1) announcing the data on which the decision is based, and (2) providing interested persons an opportunity to petition the FDA within 30 days for reconsideration of the decision.[26]

In the event of a medical device requiring further evaluation before a 510(k) premarket notification or PMA, an investigational device exemption can be applied for.[26] In this instance, any approval process is overseen by related institutional review boards in addition to the FDA. Once all criteria are met, one may proceed to distribute the device to investigators free from the FDA compliance regulations.

TEMPs

TEMPs have arisen consequent to the advent of TE and the role of nondevice interventions that fall between biomaterials and cell-based technologies. These products are often combinations of cells, scaffolds, and other factors, and are complex in both structure and function. Since the 1997 inception of Division IV of the committee F04 on Medical and Surgical Material and Devices was formed,[29] these entities have been regulated by several bodies within the FDA. The primary regulatory bodies are the Office of Combination products (OCP) and the tissue reference group (TRG).[30]

Owing to the diversity of multiple cell-based TEMPs, their regulation is still being developed and, as such, the standards process for these products is under way within the American Society for Testing and Materials International Committee F-04, Division IV Tissue Engineered Medical Products (http://www.astm.org/) of Committee F04 on Medical and Surgical Materials and Devices.[31,32]

PRODUCTION IN A GMP FACILITY

Surgeon-scientists who have successfully negotiated the development of their discovery to the point of market and manufacture must establish and follow quality systems to help ensure that their products consistently meet all applicable FDA regulations and specifications. These regulations require manufacturers to ensure that products are safe, pure, and effective.

The quality systems for FDA-regulated products are known as current good manufacturing practices (cGMPs). The FDA is revising the current cGMPs for medical devices and TEMPs, and is incorporating them into a quality system regulation. For a producer to achieve these goals (unless exempt[33]) all aspects of manufacturing should be monitored (and will be routinely inspected), including quality assurance management, personnel, premises and equipment, documentation, production, quality control, contract manufacture and analysis, complaints, and product recall.[33]

CLINICAL TRIALS
Clinical Trials with Medical Devices

To gain ultimate FDA approval by PMA, most medical devices require submission of clinical data to support claims made for the device. It is critical to appreciate that the development of a medical device or a TEMPs is very much different to that of a drug.[34]

Medical device research involves substantial bench and animal testing for reliability and biocompatibility (eg, in breast implants), but there are no studies for toxicity on devices, as opposed to the studies required for pharmaceutical research. Pilot and feasibility studies on medical devices are considered first-in-man studies with device development being iterative. Designs may be refined or improved as device development progresses.

Although user feedback, adverse events, or difficulties in deploying or delivering a device can all lead to changes to the device, second- or third-generation designs do not always require a new clinical trial. Bridging the new to the old design may require additional bench studies or small confirmatory postmarket studies. The 2 main types of study are the reproducibility study (to prove accuracy and precision) and the clinical utility study (to demonstrate real-life use of the device).

Clinical Trials with TEMPs

TEMPs are regulated by the FDA by several different pathways according to their composition. As part of the TEMPs, combination products are commonly developed by surgeon-scientists and are regulated by the OCP (http://www.fda.gov/oc/combination/CombinationProducts). Before initiating clinical trials, there are some critical considerations in commercializing a TEMP.

Although jurisdiction decisions can frequently be obtained informally for novel or complex products, there is a formal process in place for combination products based on the determination of their primary mode of action (PMOA) through which the product achieves its effect. This approach is used to determine which of the 3 centers that regulate human medical products will be the regulatory body (Center for Biologics Evaluation and Research, Center for Drug Evaluation and Research, or CDRH).

Before the initiation of any clinical studies with TEMPs, it is essential to determine the structure of the product. Many TEMPs in the current market or currently under development are products in which cells are combined with a biomaterial scaffold. The scaffold serves as a matrix that provides support for growth of new tissue. These products pose novel challenges that may have significant bearing on how clinical products are developed.

Undoubtedly, one of the biggest challenges for the inventor of a cell-scaffold combination product arises from the fact that the product will combine distinct components that are developed under different manufacturing and regulatory approaches. Furthermore, these products are not defined solely by the individual components because once the product is assembled and cell-scaffold interactions commence, the product's properties will inevitably change. Thus when evaluating cell-scaffold products, it is essential to distinguish studies that need to be conducted on individual components before assembly.

Unique to this product class is that they may not be in their active form when administered to the patient, as in vivo remodeling will occur. For this reason complete functional testing is impossible, so the product may require preclinical proof-of-concept studies and in vivo safety data to rule out any potential construct failures before clinical studies commence.

Surgeon-scientists may increase the likelihood of achieving clinical approval for TEMPs by developing and refining new product manufacturing and characterization techniques early in the process. It is advised that one should take advantage of the overabundance of informal routes of communication possible with the FDA to obtain timely and accurate feedback from the agency regarding specific products, to ensure efficient progression of new products toward clinical trials.

SUMMARY

This article attempts to provide an up-to-date overview of commercial development of a patentable discovery for aspiring hand surgeon-scientist entrepreneurs. The information provided pertains largely to researchers in the United States, but the authors trust that the information will also be helpful to clinicians worldwide.

The guide provided could also help clinicians navigate the often confounding interface between the IP law and scientific research, recognizing that models of funding scientific research are rapidly evolving and that startup development is a formidable challenge.

Finally, it is hoped that this review provides an understanding of the logistics of the patent prosecution, such that one is better informed to leverage opportunities for resources to bring basic science and innovation into daily clinical practice.

REFERENCES

1. Murphy BD, Zuker RM, Borshel GH. Vascularized composite allotransplantation: an update on medical and surgical progress and remaining challenges. J Plast Reconstr Aesthet Surg 2013;66:1449–55.
2. Piza-Katzer H, Wechselberger G, Estermann D, et al. Ten years of hand transplantation experiment or routine? Handchir Mikrochir Plast Chir 2009;41:210–6 [in German].
3. Scher R, Hautz T, Brandacher G, et al. Immunosuppression in hand transplantation: state of the art and future prospects. Handchir Mikrochir Plast Chir 2009;41:217–23 [in German].
4. Kermit EL. From concept to exit strategies-medical device innovation. Conf Proc IEEE Eng Med Biol Soc 2004;7:5130.
5. US patent statistics, Calendar years 1963-2012. Available at: http://www.uspto.gov/web/offices/ac/ido/oeip/taf/us_stat.pdf. Accessed May 19, 2014.
6. Sheiness D, Canady K. The importance of getting inventorship right. Nat Biotechnol 2006;24:153.
7. Baker S, Weinzweig J. Bioentrepreneurialism for the plastic surgeon. Plast Reconstr Surg 2008;122:295–301.

8. United States Patent and Trademark Office. AIA Resources. Available at: http://www.uspto.gov/aia_implementation/resoucres.jsp. Accessed February 11, 2013.

9. Stanford Office of Licensing and Technology. Highlights of the America Invents Act. Available at: http://otl.stanford.edu/documents/aiamemo.pdf. Accessed May 19, 2014.

10. Das OP. Building relationships with technology transfer officers. Nat Biotechnol 2005;23:781.

11. Roberts MJ. The legal protection of intellectual property. April 17, 1998. From lecture ordered as reprint from HBR reprint number 9-898-230.

12. Gautam G, Abhijit G, Spencer R, et al. Evaluation of a novel connexin-based peptide for the treatment of diabetic wounds. The 2013 ASCI/AAP Joint Meeting. Chicago, IL, April 26–28, 2008. [abstract 190].

13. Aldag J, Kessel M, Ibrahim A, et al. Other ways of financing your company. Nat Biotechnol 2008; 26(2):1–3.

14. Mullen P. Where VC fears to tread. Biotechnol Healthc 2007;4(5):29–35.

15. Burns LR, Housman MG, Robinson CA. Market entry and exit by biotech and device companies funded by venture capital. Health Aff 2009;28(1): w76–86.

16. Lazonick W, Tulum Ö. US biopharmaceutical finance and the sustainability of the biotech boom. Industry Studies Working Paper: 2010-01. 2010. Available at: http://www.nextnewdeal.net/wp-content/uploads/2011/07/biopharmaceutical-finance.pdf. Accessed May 19, 2014.

17. Elsbach K. How to pitch a brilliant idea. Harv Bus Rev 2003;81:117–23.

18. Boezi K, Parks E, Shawver L. Power dating: a guide to VC courtship. Nat Biotechnol 2006;24:895.

19. Zider B. How venture capital works. Harv Bus Rev 1998;76:131–9.

20. Roberts MJ. How venture capitalists evaluate potential venture opportunities. Harv Bus Rev 2004;17:289–333.

21. Beyond borders: global biotechnology report. 2011. Available at: http://www.ey.com/GL/en/Industries/Life-Sciences/Beyond-borders-globalbiotechnology-report-2011. Accessed November 16, 2013.

22. Ben-Menachem G. Doing business with the NIH. Nat Biotechnol 2006;24:17.

23. The Angel Investor Market Q1Q2 2013 report. Available at: https://paulcollege.unh.edu/sites/paulcollege.unh.edu/files/Q1Q2%202013%20Analysis%20Report.pdf. Accessed November 16, 2013.

24. FDA: implants and prosthetics. Available at: http://www.fda.gov/MedicalDevices/ProductsandMedicalProcedures/ImplantsandProsthetics/Referenced. Accessed October 21, 2013.

25. FDA: medical devices: overview of device regulation. Available at: http://www.fda.gov/MedicalDevices/DeviceRegulationandGuidance/Overview/default.htm. Accessed May 19, 2014.

26. FDA: medical devices: device advice: Investigational Device Exemption (IDE). Available at: http://www.fda.gov/MedicalDevices/DeviceRegulationandGuidance/HowtoMarketYourDevice/InvestigationalDeviceExemptionIDE/. Accessed May 19, 2014.

27. FDA: medical devices: Premarket notification (510k). Available at: http://www.fda.gov/medicaldevices/deviceregulationandguidance/howtomarketyourdevice/premarketsubmissions/premarketnotification510k/default.htm. Accessed May 19, 2014.

28. FDA: medical devices: Premarket approval. Available at: http://www.fda.gov/medicaldevices/deviceregulationandguidance/howtomarketyourdevice/premarketsubmissions/premarketapprovalpma/. Accessed May 19, 2014.

29. Piccolo GL, Hellman KB, Johnson PC. Meeting report: tissue engineered medical products standards: the time is ripe. Tissue Eng 1998;4:5–7. Available at: http://www.fda.gov/MedicalDevices/DeviceRegulationandGuidance/Standards/ucm135382.htm.

30. FDA: vaccines, blood and biologics: Tissue Reference Group. Available at: http://www.fda.gov/biologicsbloodvaccines/tissuetissueproducts/regulationoftissues/ucm152857.htm. Accessed May 19, 2014.

31. FDA: Tissue Engineered Medical Products Standards (TEMPS). Available at: http://www.fda.gov/MedicalDevices/DeviceRegulationandGuidance/Standards/ucm135369.htm. Accessed May 19, 2014.

32. FDA: medical device exemptions 510(k) and GMP requirements. Available at: http://www.accessdata.fda.gov/scripts/cdrh/cfdocs/cfpcd/315.cfm. Accessed May 19, 2014.

33. FDA: medical devices: Current Good Manufacturing (cGMP) Final Rule; Quality System regulation. Available at: http://www.fda.gov/medicaldevices/deviceregulationandguidance/postmarketrequirements/qualitystsyemsregulations/ucm230127.htm. Accessed January 11, 2013.

34. Campbell G. The role of statistics in medical devices - the contrast with pharmaceuticals. Biopharmaceutical Report 2006;14:1–8.

Comparative Effectiveness Research in Hand Surgery

Shepard P. Johnson, MBBS[a], Kevin C. Chung, MD, MS[b],*

KEYWORDS

- Comparative effectiveness research • Hand surgery • Large databases
- Patient-reported outcomes

KEY POINTS

- The US Institute of Medicine in 2008 started a national initiative of research known as comparative effectiveness research (CER), which will support better decision making about interventions in health care.
- CER focuses on interventions that occur within real-world environments, therefore the conclusions can be generalized to a broad population.
- CER conducted through large electronic databases allows researchers to evaluate how current health care practices affect the outcomes of care.
- To date, there is minimal comparative effectiveness evidence in hand surgery, which is partly attributed to the lack of relevant outcomes information included in electronic databases.
- Inclusion of patient-related outcomes into electronic databases will facilitate the adaptation of CER into hand surgery.

INTRODUCTION

The US Institute of Medicine (IOM) in 2008 started a national initiative known comparative effectiveness research (CER) to support better decision making about interventions in medicine.[1] Clinical decision making varies based on patient factors, clinicians' experience, and regional preferences. These decisions are often made without supportive evidence. Inconsistent clinical practice is well recognized and raises concerns about the appropriateness and economics of current medicine, which is evident from the cost and outcome differences that exist in health care across the United States.[2] The IOM attributes inconsistencies in health care delivery to the lack of information available to make well-informed decisions in everyday clinical medicine.

The IOM publicized the need for high-impact research to improve the quality and efficiency of health care in a comprehensive report in 2008.[3] In response, legislators passed the American Recovery and Reinvestment Act (ARRA) of 2009, which allocated $1.1 billion to fund CER.[1] The Federal Coordinating Council and an appointed IOM committee were charged with identifying high-priority research topics and to allocate funds from the ARRA. The President distributed these funds to the National Institutes of Health (NIH), Agency for Health Research and Quality (AHRQ), and Office of the Secretary of the US Department of Health

Supported in part by grants from the National Institute of Arthritis and Musculoskeletal and Skin Diseases (2R01AR047328 - 06, R01 AR062066) and a Midcareer Investigator Award in Patient-Oriented Research (2K24-AR053120-06) to Dr. Kevin C. Chung.

[a] Department of Surgery, Saint Joseph Mercy Hospital, 5333 McAuley Drive, Reichert Health Building, Suite R-2111, Ann Arbor, MI 48197, USA; [b] Section of Plastic Surgery, Faculty Affairs, University of Michigan Health System, University of Michigan Medical School, 2130 Taubman Center, SPC 5340, 1500 East Medical Center Drive, Ann Arbor, MI 48109-5340, USA

* Corresponding author.
E-mail address: kecchung@umich.edu

Hand Clin 30 (2014) 319–327
http://dx.doi.org/10.1016/j.hcl.2014.04.001
0749-0712/14/$ – see front matter © 2014 Elsevier Inc. All rights reserved.

and Human Services (DHHS). In 2010, as part of the Affordable Care Act, legislators established an ongoing national program in CER, the Patient-Centered Outcomes Research Institute (PCORI).[4]

CER is not a novel concept, but represents a research movement propagated by a large investment by the federal government. CER can be conceptualized as a form of outcomes research. This research asks which intervention is most effective, for whom, and under what circumstances.[5] Through encouragement from the IOM, CER trials often use large electronic databases to study current health practices and outcomes. They are often referred to as pragmatic trials, because they reflect routine clinical practice.[6]

Hand surgery has embraced outcomes research and, to better evaluate effectiveness of interventions, have developed questionnaires such as the Michigan Hand Outcomes Questionnaire (MHQ). The MHQ is a subjective evaluation tool used to measure outcomes such as hand function and pain.[7] These instruments report patient-related outcomes (PROs), a recognized and standardized method of reporting patients' perspectives on interventions.[8] PROs provide the patients' perspectives on treatment benefit and can be the outcome of greatest importance.[8] Therefore, incorporating PROs into CER greatly enhances the quality of hand surgery research, thus providing better evidence on which to base clinical decisions.

DEFINITION OF CER

CER is designed to provide information about the relative effectiveness of different medical interventions to improve the quality and value of care.[9] The IOM defines CER as "the generation and synthesis of evidence that compares the benefits and harms of alternative methods to prevent, diagnose, treat, and monitor a clinical condition or to improve the delivery of care."[3] When conducting CER, investigators are asking themselves how an intervention compares, both overall and in subsets of the population.[10] Therefore, researchers seek to determine what interventions are appropriate for particular patients and populations within a variety of circumstances. CER investigates interventions, tests (eg, diagnostic, therapeutic), prevention strategies, care delivery, and quality of care.[4]

The IOM adds that "...the purpose of CER is to assist consumers, clinicians, purchasers, and policy makers to make informed decisions that will improve health care at both the individual and population level."[8] Thus, information should lead to more standardized care, and should recognize that decisions may vary if individuals are categorized in a particular subset. The IOM clearly identifies multiple stakeholders, outside the doctor-patient relationship, including payers and policy makers. In acknowledging these stakeholders, there is an underlying national objective of optimizing health outcomes within financial and resource constraints.[11]

METHODOLOGY OF CER

CER is the study of 2 different but accepted standard practices, neither of which is superior based on available medical evidence.[6] Interventions are simple and occur within practical clinical settings. A key component is the use of real-world data, therefore reflecting patients who are typical of day-to-day clinical care.[1] Without specific patient inclusion criteria, conclusions are drawn from a population representative of those who would receive the intervention in a normal clinical setting.[9] Observational CER studies include patient cohorts numbering in the thousands that are achieved through large medical databases. Outcomes of CER studies are intended to be clinically relevant, meaningful to the patient and general public, and subject to minimal ascertainment bias.[4,12]

CER methodologies are in contrast with classical double-blinded randomized controlled trials (RCTs), which are conducted on highly selected populations with rigorous inclusion and exclusion criteria. Study enrollment in RCTs includes patients with few comorbidities in order to optimize statistical power and the benefit/risk trade-off.[11] These so-called efficacy studies assess whether an intervention is efficacious under ideal, controlled settings.[1,11] The outcome measures of efficacy trials are often arbitrary and less clinically relevant.[6] RCTs answer the question "does this work?"[1] Alternatively, CER provides decision makers with the answer to "is this better than that?."[1] In simplistic terms, CER studies are less controlled, with fewer exclusion criteria, and therefore the conclusions can be generalized to a large population. The IOM supports the broad use of evidence to evaluate effectiveness,[11] including systematic reviews, retrospective database analysis, prospective observational studies, or pragmatic RCTs. Despite this statement, there is strong emphasis placed on observational, database research. **Table 1** shows the characteristic differences between classic RCTs and observational, database-conducted CER.

THE VALUE OF ELECTRONIC DATABASES IN CER

Electronic databases, including administrative claims databases and electronic health record

Table 1
A characteristic comparison of observational, database CER, and classic multi-institutional RCTs

	Conventional RCTs	Database CER
Design	**Interventional**	**Observational**
Patients/population	Patients with few comorbidities	Patients represent those typically seen in everyday practice
	Rigorous inclusion/exclusion criteria	Minimal inclusion/exclusion criteria
Intervention	Intervention of interest	An acceptable standard of practice
Control	Placebo or standard of practice	Alternative acceptable standard(s) of practice
Outcome	Does this work? Is the intervention efficacious in the highly selected population? Composite end point (eg, improved range of motion)	Is this better than that? Is the intervention effective in the general population? Outcomes meaningful to patient/public (eg, PRO)
Study size	Hundreds	Thousands
Data collection	Single, multiple institution sites	Electronic medical records/databases
Study of population subsets	Difficult	Possible (encouraged by the IOM)
Duration	Long	Short
Cost	Expensive	Low cost per patient
Bias	Selection bias/confounding minimized in double-blinded studies	Selection, indication bias problematic

databases, allow researchers to evaluate how current health care practices affect the outcome of care.[1] The IOM understands that the success of CER depends on the quality of electronic clinical data. They recommend that "The CER Program should help to develop large-scale, clinical and administrative data networks to facilitate better use of data and more efficient ways to collect new data to yield CER findings."[3] This recommendation applies particularly to hand surgery, in which subjective outcomes such as pain and aesthetics are critical in evaluating intervention effectiveness.[5] At present, databases do not routinely collect this information.[13]

In using large electronic databases, observational research can be fast, low cost, high volume, and can represent real-world decisions.[1] In addition, large-scale observational studies may confirm results of randomized trials in understudied patient subsets, inform about rare events, and provide insight into the processes of care delivery.[14] Databases allow subgroup analysis and assessment of treatment heterogeneity. Identification of characteristics among subgroups may help to identify key predictors of response.[1] Individual responses to health interventions must not be overlooked, because subsets of populations may have very different responses to interventions compared with the whole population.[14] Individual differences

may include genetic risk factors and environmental exposures.

Making accurate inferences from observational studies can be challenging. Therefore, the AHRQ has helped to develop the Electronic Data Methods (EDM) forum to advance the knowledge and practice of the use of electronic clinical data for CER.[15] Critical issues that this organization addresses include confounding adjustment approaches for observational CER studies, models for evaluating data variability and quality, patient privacy and data security, and incorporating PROs into CER.[15]

The Healthcare Cost and Utilization Project (HCUP), a collection of electronic databases and software tools, is an example of a database that could be used in hand CER studies.[13,16] Data collected within HCUP include international classification of disease diagnosis codes, demographic information, cost of stay, length of stay, and other administrative information.[13] However, drawing conclusions about the effectiveness of interventions, such as patients with rheumatoid arthritis who have undergone arthrodesis, is difficult with this information. Unlike other surgical specialties, outcomes such as length of stay, readmission rates, mortality, or major clinical events (eg, myocardial infarction) are less common in hand surgery. Outcomes pertinent to a patient considering arthrodesis include functionality, pain, return to work, aesthetics, and ability to perform activities of daily living.[5] PRO questionnaires, such as the MHQ, provide a reliable and efficient way to document these outcomes. Creating databases that contain this information is necessary to make assessments of effectiveness for hand surgical interventions.

Table 2 lists CER studies from a range of specialties that have used large databases to conduct observational research. Note the various electronic databases that are used, including administrative, specialty specific, Medicare, and Medicaid. When designing a CER study in hand surgery, selecting the appropriate database is imperative. **Fig. 1** shows important database characteristics that facilitate a well-conducted study. They should include accurate and uniform documentation of patient demographics, diagnoses, and outcomes.

INCORPORATING PROS INTO CER

To provide sufficient informed decision making, CER studies should seek to measure all outcomes that are important to patients.[9] Conventional end points, such as disease-free interval, do not provide consumers with a complete understanding of treatment effects. PROs are any reports coming directly from patients about how they function or feel in relation to a health condition and its therapy.[17] Constructs that can be assessed with PROs include symptoms, functional status, health-related quality of life (HRQoL), health behaviors, and patient satisfaction with care.[18] For example, HRQoL measures include perceptions about health in general, physical function, social functioning, and psychological well-being.[19] A study by Waljee and colleagues[20] showed that the MHQ, which measures several HRQoL constructs, is an essential instrument for understanding the extent of disability of rheumatic hand disease. These outcomes are best judged by patients and they define effectiveness in a way that clinical measures (eg, blood pressure, laboratory tests) cannot.[19]

Measuring PROs can be accomplished through structured questionnaires or interviews. These subjective measurement tools should ideally be easy to administer, quick, and low cost. The quality of an instrument is based on its clinimetric properties, which include reliability, validity, responsiveness, and interpretability.[8,21] The MHQ, a PRO questionnaire, is one such instrument that has proved to be responsive in evaluating outcomes in a variety of conditions related to the hand.[5] Waljee and colleagues[20] showed that the MHQ is easily administered, reliable, and valid in measuring

rheumatoid hand function, thus providing a clinical way to measure outcomes in rheumatic hand disease. The MHQ is also responsive in measuring outcomes involving distal radius fractures.[22] A separate subjective assessment tool, the Carpal Tunnel Questionnaire, has been shown to have greater responsiveness to clinical change following carpal tunnel repair than the MHQ.[23] Therefore, the most appropriate PRO tool may vary based on the hand condition of interest.

PCORI, a nonprofit corporation, was established in 2010 by the Patient Protection and Affordable Care Act (ACA) and has promoted patient-centered outcomes research (PCOR). PCOR, a branch of CER, is primarily intended to inform decision making among individual patients. To accomplish this, PCOR focuses on outcomes "that people notice and care about such as survival, function, symptoms and HRQoL."[24] PCOR emphasizes the patient perspective and supports the inclusion of PROs within CER.[24,25] Hand research has already widely adapted subjective assessment tools. Promoting the inclusion of questionnaires, such as the MHQ, into electronic databases would be a substantial advancement toward CER in hand surgery.

Snyder and colleagues[25] identified several practical issues/challenges to the incorporation of PROs into PCOR, including the comprehensive and uniform adoption of PROs, the proprietary nature of the measurement tools, selection of the best PRO, and the clinical interpretation of PROs.[25] At an institutional level, PRO tools are often used by individual investigators or research groups. Standardizing and integrating PRO tools into clinical practice across the country would take considerable effort and possibly governance policy.[25] Snyder and colleagues[25] postulated that, perhaps in the future, a PRO test may be billable to insurers, much as laboratory tests are. Uniform use of PRO tools and the incorporation of these data into electronic health records/databases will take a concerted effort to establish.

EFFECTIVENESS STUDIES IN HAND SURGERY

To date, there have been minimal CER studies, federally or privately funded, on interventions within hand surgery. The CER Database, maintained by the National Patient Advocate Foundation (NPAF), compiles comparative studies funded by the NIH and AHRQ (http://www.npaf.org).[26] The CER Inventory provides an inventory of projects funded by agencies within the DHHS (http://cerdatatracker.org/).[27] Within these inventories there are multiple trials studying the biological and nonsurgical therapies for rheumatoid

Table 2
Examples of CER studies that used observational database methodologies

Author	Topic	Database Study Size (N)	Outcomes Measured	Investigators' Conclusions
Dewitt et al,[31] 2013	Nonbiologic vs biologic DMARDs for RA treatment	US-based observational registry (2001–2008) N = 1729	CDAI scores	Both treatment groups experienced lower CDAI scores across time. Patients switching to DMARD showed greater improvement than patients switching to nonbiologic DMARD
Grijalva et al,[32] 2008	Patterns of medication use in RA	Tennessee Medicaid (1995–2004) N = 23,342	Patterns of DMARD use	The use of DMARDs increased in TennCare patients with RA, and, by 2004, use of biologics was substantial. Although glucocorticoid use decreased, use of both NSAIDs and narcotics increased
Solomon et al,[33] 2010	Comparative safety of opioids	Medicare (1996–2005) N = 6275	Cardiovascular events, factures, gastrointestinal events	The rates of safety events among elderly adults using opioids for nonmalignant pain vary significantly by agent
McCutcheon et al,[34] 2013	Surgeons vs interventionalists in performing EVAR	Nationwide inpatient sample (1998–2009) N = 28,094	Mortality, length of stay, hospital charge	Surgeons are associated with improved outcomes, lower mortality, shorter length of stay, and lower charges for EVAR cases, compared with interventionalists
Martin et al,[35] 2011	Three oral bisphosphonates	Administrative claims databases (2005–2007) N = 45,939	Fractures, time to fracture, health care cost	Rates of adherence and total adjusted all-cause health care costs for alendronate, risedronate, and ibandronate are similar. Absolute, unadjusted rates of fracture were small and did not significantly differ among agents
Aghayev et al,[36] 2012	Lumbar TDA vs ALIF	SWISSspine registry (2005–2010) N = 534	QoL, pain alleviation	Pain alleviation after TDA and ALIF was similar
Eurich et al,[37] 2013	Sitagliptin vs other glucose-lowering agents in type 2 diabetes	US claims and integrated laboratory databases[a] (2004–2009) N = 72,738	Hospital admissions, mortality	Sitagliptin use was not associated with an excess risk of all-cause hospital admission or death compared with other glucose-lowering agents

Abbreviations: ALIF, anterior lumbar interbody fusion; CDAI, Clinical Disease Activity Index; DMARD, disease-modifying antirheumatic drugs; EVAR, endovascular aortic aneurysm repair; NSAIDs, nonsteroidal antiinflammatory drugs; QoL, quality of life; RA, rheumatoid arthritis; TDA, total disc arthroplasty.
[a] Clinformatics DATA Mart, OptumInsight Life Sciences Inc.

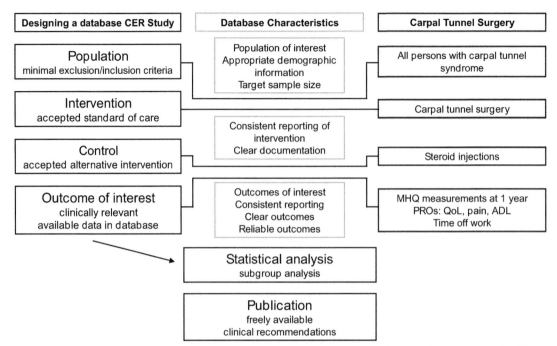

Fig. 1. Selecting the appropriate database is critical in designing observational CER studies. Column 2 highlights important database characteristics. Column 3 offers an example within hand surgery. ADL, activities of daily living; QoL, quality of life.

arthritis, osteoarthritis, and osteoporosis, but there is only 1 publication directly related to the comparative effectiveness of a hand topic. This is an ARRA-funded study titled The Value of High Quality Medical Care for Work-associated Carpal Tunnel Syndrome (Steven Asch, Rand Corporation) scheduled to be completed by 7/31/2015.[26] **Table 3** lists ongoing studies funded by federal grants from the NIH and ARHQ as listed on the NPAF Web site[26] that relate to the musculoskeletal system.

In addition to the federal investment in the national CER program, the private sector is equally important in supporting effectiveness research. None of the original high-priority topics identified by the IOM (which received most of the ARRA funding) were directly relevant to hand surgery interventions.[2] At present, there seems to be minimal CER concerning the hand. A basic search for the term comparative effectiveness in PubMed fails to identify large-scale database-conducted observational trials related to carpal tunnel syndrome. A cosearch of comparative effectiveness and radial fracture (or distal radial fracture) identifies 1 large database study by Chung and colleagues.[28] They performed an analysis of Medicare data to evaluate the variations in the use of internal fixation for distal radial fractures in the United States. They found that the use of internal

fixation differs widely across geographic regions. The investigators concluded that the variation in treatment was a result of the lack of comparative effectiveness evidence.[28]

Although this study did not directly compare two interventions, or determine effectiveness of internal fixation of radial fracture, it highlights an obstacle in database research within hand surgery. Their conclusions were drawn from limited data, including basic patient demographics, comorbidities, presence of osteoporosis, concurrent ulnar fracture, type of surgeon, and geographic information.[28] As mentioned previously, evaluating effectiveness of interventions requires information on outcomes such as pain, functionality, and aesthetics.

CHALLENGES IN CER

"CER is as vulnerable to bias and conflict of interest as any other area of medical research."[1] By emphasizing observational studies, with limited exclusion criteria, CER is particularly susceptible to selection and indication bias.[29] Selection bias refers to systematic differences between baseline characteristics of the groups that are compared.[17] Indication bias is also referred to as confounding by indication and confounding by severity of disease. Characteristics of patients that dictate clinical

Table 3
Federal grants for musculoskeletal-related comparative effectiveness studies funded by the NIH and AHRQ as listed on the NPAF Web site (http://www.npaf.org/news/CER-database-launched)

Primary Investigator	Grant Number	Topic	Database	Outcomes	Project End
Asch, Steven M. (RAND Corporation)	R01 HS18982-01	Work-associated CTS	Compensation claims in northern California	Quality of medical care measured by RAND/UCLA CTS quality measures	07/31/2015
Bannuru, Raveendhara (Tufts Medical Center)	F32 HS21396-01A1	Medical treatments for knee osteoarthritis	Unspecified (planned network meta-analysis)	Unspecified	06/30/2013
Saag, Kenneth (University of Alabama at Birmingham)	U19 HS21110-01	Multiple NSAIDs vs narcotics after joint replacement surgery	Unspecified	Unspecified	08/31/2016
Tosteson, Anna (Dartmouth College)	R01 HS18405-01	Treatments for degenerative spine disease	Medicare claims and SPORT	Unspecified	01/31/2013

Abbreviations: CTS, carpal tunnel syndrome; SPORT, Spine Patient Outcomes Research Trial; UCLA, University of California, Los Angeles.
Data from NPAF. National Patient Advocate Foundation launches Comparative Effectiveness Research (CER) database. Available at: http://www.npaf.org/news/CER-database-launched. Accessed October 9, 2013.

decisions may influence outcomes, prompting debate on whether the intervention or the patient determines the outcome[1]; this is an example of confounding by indication. Confounders may also arise at an institutional level if different treatment preferences or reimbursement policies exist.[30] Statisticians attempt to correct for indication bias through adjustments with disease severity scoring systems or propensity scores, but the only way to eliminate it is through randomization.[28] In IOM's 2009 sentinel article, they acknowledge that "overcoming the limitations of observational research is the most important frontier of research on study methods."[2]

Improving clinical decision making will depend on the results of CER studies. Therefore, a premium should be placed on identifying the most pertinent outcomes to measure. Because the definition of CER identifies multiple stakeholders, the outcomes of greatest importance may vary.[29] Furthermore, what constitutes a benefit will vary among these stakeholders. For example, patients may base decisions on pain relief from carpal tunnel syndrome, whereas a policy maker or payers may place an emphasis on cost of care or time to return to work.

By providing quality evidence of effectiveness, CER will theoretically reduce variation in care and minimize unnecessary, costly interventions,[9] and this is the justification behind the federal funding. The explicit exclusion of cost-effectiveness analysis (CEA) remains a controversial topic. CEA in countries such as Australia, the United Kingdom, and Canada plays an integral role in the development of clinical guidelines,[11] which aids in determining the greatest health benefit within a limited budget.[9] CEA is intentionally excluded by the ACA, which prohibits PCORI from engaging in research measuring value of interventions.[9] Those opposing CEA within CER argue that the federal government should not participate in cost considerations in research. This argument is considered to be rationing and governmental interference in patient care. Because PCORI is an integral part of CER, Garber and Sox[9] think that it should continue to collect data on cost, which would allow private analysts to conduct research that provides important cost outcomes information.[9]

SUMMARY

The national movement to conduct CER is in response to the lack of information that exists to make evidence-based clinical decisions. The IOM thinks that, through showing the effectiveness of alternative treatments, patients and other stakeholders will be equipped with the knowledge to choose the appropriate treatment. The federal government has demonstrated its commitment to this research through funding and the establishment of organizations, such as PCORI. Although surgical interventions in the hand were not among the high-priority topics identified by the IOM in 2008, this movement presents an opportunity to participate in robust database research. For hand surgeons to benefit from electronic health databases, they should promote the incorporation of outcomes data that are relevant to surgical interventions. This incorporation can be accomplished through the inclusion of subjective measuring assessments that evaluate PROs such as pain, functionality, aesthetics, and other HRQoL measures.

REFERENCES

1. Sox HC, Greenfield S. Comparative effectiveness research: a report from the Institute of Medicine. Ann Intern Med 2009;151:203–5.
2. Ratner R, Eden J, Wolman D, et al. Initial national priorities for comparative effectiveness research. Washington, DC: National Academics Press; 2009.
3. Federal Coordinating Council for Comparative Effectiveness Research. Report to the President and Congress. Washington, DC: Department of Health and Human Services; 2009.
4. Sox HC. Comparative effectiveness research: a progress report. Ann Intern Med 2010;153:469–72.
5. Chung KC. Clinical research in hand surgery. J Hand Surg 2010;35:109–20.
6. Klein HG. Comparative effectiveness research: welcome to the real world. Transfusion 2012;52:1162–4.
7. Chung KC, Pillsbury MS, Walters MR, et al. Reliability and validity testing of the Michigan Hand Outcomes Questionnaire. J Hand Surg 1998;23:575–87.
8. van der Wal M, Verhaegen P, Middelkoop E, et al. A clinimetric overview of scar assessment scales. J Burn Care Res 2012;33:e79–87.
9. Garber AM, Sox HC. The role of costs in comparative effectiveness research. Health Aff (Millwood) 2010;29:1805–11.
10. Temple R. A regulator's view of comparative effectiveness research. Clin Trials 2012;9:56–65.
11. Goss CH, Tefft N. Comparative effectiveness research - what is it and how does one do it? Paediatr Respir Rev 2013;14:152–6.
12. Sox HC, Helfand M, Grimshaw J, et al. Comparative effectiveness research: challenges for medical journals. Trials 2010;11:45.
13. HCUP. Overview of HCUP. Available at: http://www.hcup-us.ahrq.gov/overview.jsp. Accessed October 4, 2012.
14. Lauer MS, Collins FS. Using science to improve the nation's health system: NIH's commitment to

comparative effectiveness research. JAMA 2010; 303:2182–3.

15. Holve E, Calonge N. Lessons from the electronic data methods forum. Med Care 2013;51:S1–3.

16. Malay S, Shauver MJ, Chung KC. Applicability of large databases in outcomes research. J Hand Surg Am 2012;37:1437–46.

17. Higgins JP, Green S. Cochrane handbook for systematic reviews of interventions version 5.1.0 [updated March 2011]. The Cochrane Collaboration. Available at: www.cochrane-handbook.org. Accessed October 9, 2013.

18. Ahmed S, Berzon RA, Revicki DA, et al. The use of patient-reported outcomes (PRO) within comparative effectiveness research: implications for clinical practice and health care policy. Med Care 2012; 50:1060–70.

19. Wu AB, Snyder C, Clancy CM, et al. Adding the patient perspective to comparative effectiveness research. Health Aff 2010;29:1863–70.

20. Waljee JF, Chung KC, Kim HM, et al. Validity and responsiveness of the Michigan Hand Questionnaire in patients with rheumatoid arthritis: a multicenter, international study. Arthritis Care Res 2010;62:1569–77.

21. Tyack Z, Simons M, Spinks A, et al. A systematic review of the quality of burn scar rating scales for clinical and research use. Burns 2012;38:6–18.

22. Kotsis SV, Lau FH, Chung KC. Responsiveness of the Michigan Hand Outcomes Questionnaire and physical measurements in outcome studies of distal radius fracture treatment. J Hand Surg Am 2007;32: 84–90.

23. Chatterjee JS, Price PE. Comparative responsiveness of the Michigan Hand Outcomes Questionnaire and the Carpal Tunnel Questionnaire after carpal tunnel release. J Hand Surg 2009;34:273–80.

24. D'Arcy LP, Rich EC. From comparative effectiveness research to patient-centered outcomes research: policy history and future directions. Neurosurg Focus 2012;33:E7,. 1–5.

25. Snyder CF, Jensen RE, Segal JB, et al. Patient-reported outcomes (PROs): putting the patient perspective in patient-centered outcomes research. Med Care 2013;51:S73–9.

26. NPAF. National Patient Advocate Foundation launches Comparative Effectiveness Research (CER) database. Available at: http://www.npaf.org/news/CER-database-launched. Accessed October 9, 2013.

27. HHS/PIPC. Comparative effectiveness research inventory. Available at: http://cerdatatracker.org. Accessed October 9, 2013.

28. Chung KC, Shauver MJ, Huiying Y, et al. Variations in the use of internal fixation for distal radial fracture in the United States Medicare population. J Bone Joint Surg Am 2011;93:2154–62.

29. Goss CH. Comparative effectiveness research: what happened to incorporating costs of care? Am J Respir Crit Care Med 2011;183:973–4.

30. Toh S, Gagne JJ, Rassen JA, et al. Confounding adjustments in comparative effectiveness research conducted within distributed research networks. Med Care 2013;51:S1–10.

31. Dewitt EM, Li Y, Curtis JR, et al. Comparative effectiveness of nonbiologic versus biologic disease-modifying antirheumatic drugs for rheumatoid arthritis. J Rheumatol 2013;40(2):127–36.

32. Grijalva CG, Chung CP, Stein CM, et al. Changing patterns of medication use in patients with rheumatoid arthritis in a Medicaid population. Rheumatology (Oxford) 2008;47(7):1061–4.

33. Solomon DH, Rassen JA, Glynn RJ, et al. The comparative safety of opioids for nonmalignant pain in older patients. Arch Intern Med 2010; 170(22):1979–86.

34. McCutcheon BA, Talamnini MA, Chang DC, et al. The comparative effectiveness of surgeons over interventionalists in endovascular repairs of abdominal aortic aneurysm. Ann Surg 2013;258(30): 476–82.

35. Martin KE, Yu J, Cambell HE, et al. Analysis of the comparative effectiveness of 3 oral bisphosphonates in a large managed care organization: adherence, fracture rates, and all-cause cost. J Manag Care Pharm 2011;17(8):596–609.

36. Aghayev E, Henning J, Munting E, et al. Comparative effectiveness research across two spine registries. Eur Spine J 2012;21(8):1640–7.

37. Eurich DT, Simpson S, Senthilselvan A, et al. Comparative safety and effectiveness of sitagliptin in patients with type 2 diabetes: retrospective population based cohort study. BMJ 2013;346: f2267.

Quality Assessment in Hand Surgery

Jennifer F. Waljee, MD, MS, MPH[a], Catherine Curtin, MD[b],*

KEYWORDS

- Hand • Surgery • Quality • Assessment

KEY POINTS

- Quality assessment and improvement is central to value-based care in the United States.
- Large payers and purchasers have incentivized quality assessment and improvement by linking reimbursement to quality metrics.
- It is critical for surgeons to understand the essential elements of quality (safety, outcomes, satisfaction, and cost) in order to optimize quality assessment and improvement efforts in hand surgery.

The quality of medical care delivered in the United States varies widely and remains difficult to define and measure. Quality assessment metrics are poorly understood for many surgical subspecialties. Nonetheless, accelerating health care costs have focused attention on ensuring quality of care for each patient, and that value is achieved with each health care dollar spent. Thus strategies to measure and optimize quality remain important for all clinicians in practice.

Quality metrics are increasingly transparent and patients now have direct access to hospital and physician metrics. Individual patient experiences are frequently presented as online on consumer blogs and search engines, and the US Centers for Medicare and Medicaid Services (CMS) allow direct comparisons of quality indicators between hospitals using the Hospital Compare website.[1] Large payers are also interested in value-based health care. For example, the CMS has instituted several programs linking reimbursement to quality metrics, such as readmission or specific complication event rates. Thus hand surgeons need to understand quality of care and its assessment not only for improving patient care but also to ensure financial and practice success.

Hand disability presents a unique challenge for those seeking to understand quality of health care. Traditional indicators, such as mortality, are not frequent enough to meaningfully measure variations in quality.[2] Thus for hand surgery 4 main areas seem to encompass most of quality of care: safety, outcomes, satisfaction, and cost. This article reviews each of these subdivisions and discusses each area's available assessment measures.

SAFETY

Since the Institute of Medicine released its landmark report *To Err is Human*, patient safety has remained at the forefront of health care policy initiatives.[3] This report highlighted the large impact of medical errors and led to standardized patient safety measures and the integration of national benchmarks to protect vulnerable patient populations. For example, there have been initiatives to reduce major inpatient perioperative complications such as perioperative deep vein thrombosis and surgical site infection. In addition, CMS defined several serious adverse events as never events (patient falls, retained foreign objects, and pressure ulcers). If never events occur, CMS has linked reduced or eliminated reimbursements.

The scope of surgical safety is enormous. Millions of Americans undergo surgery each year in the United States, accounting for approximately

[a] Section of Plastic Surgery, Department of Surgery, University of Michigan Medical Center, 1500 East Medical Center Drive, Ann Arbor, MI 48103, USA; [b] Department of Surgery, Palo Alto Veterans Hospital, 3801 Miranda Avenue, Palo Alto, CA 94304, USA
* Corresponding author.
E-mail address: curtincatherine@yahoo.com

Hand Clin 30 (2014) 329–334
http://dx.doi.org/10.1016/j.hcl.2014.04.009
0749-0712/14/$ – see front matter Published by Elsevier Inc.

40% of national health care spending.[4-6] More than 50,000 Americans die each year as a direct consequence of surgery and many more have major postoperative complications such as myocardial infarction.[7] Although surgery is becoming increasingly safe, there is substantial room for improvement.[8-10] To this end, professional organizations with federal support have developed several initiatives to measure and improve the quality of surgical care in the United States. For example, in 1991, the Veteran's Administration began prospectively following risk-adjusted surgical mortality and morbidity results.[11-14] From this effort, the National Surgical Quality Improvement Program (NSQIP) created a similar program for all hospitals, and is maintained under the auspices of the American College of Surgeons.[15,16] Using trained data abstractors, medical records are prospectively reviewed for complication rates, length of stay, perioperative mortality, and processes of care. After adjusting for case mix, risk-adjusted measures of morbidity and mortality and estimates of surgical quality can be extrapolated for participating hospitals. This methodology allows blinded comparisons between peer hospitals and merging of large numbers of cases to establish baseline rates of adverse events.[17] NSQIP has mainly been used to assess large inpatient surgeries, but is less applicable for generally safe ambulatory procedures.[18]

In the ambulatory setting, safety assessment and improvement remains more elusive. The fast pace of outpatient surgery centers raises unique patient safety concerns including correct identification of the patients and sites and ensuring that sedation is appropriate and safe. CMS has recognized these challenges and has developed a targeted set of quality measures for the ambulatory surgery setting that are now linked with reimbursement for services (**Table 1**).[19] Although ambulatory surgery safety has not yet reached the scrutiny or measurement of inpatient surgical procedures, there is increasing interest in additional assessments of outpatient surgical safety and providers need to follow closely these emerging safety measures.

OUTCOMES

Understanding patient outcomes, specifically upper extremity function and disability, is the cornerstone to capturing health care quality in hand surgery. Measures to assess functional outcomes following hand surgery are better defined than patient safety measures. Pinch and grip strength and range of motion are commonly used, are easily captured at the bedside by clinicians and therapists, and are helpful metrics of functional recovery after hand surgery.[20] These simple empirical measures of physical function do not fully capture patients' function after hand surgery. A patient with excellent grip strength but a lack of dexterity may not be able to accomplish simple everyday tasks, such as buttoning, manipulating utensils, or typing. The fuller picture of function can often be found by measuring the patient's

Table 1
CMS ambulatory surgery quality measures

Measures 2014 Payment Determination	Measures 2015 Payment Determination	Measures 2016 Payment Determination
Patient burn	Patient burn	Patient burn
Patient fall	Patient fall	Patient fall
Wrong site, wrong side, wrong patient, wrong procedure, wrong implant	Wrong site, wrong side, wrong patient, wrong procedure, wrong implant	Wrong site, wrong side, wrong patient, wrong procedure, wrong implant
Hospital transfer/admission	Hospital transfer/admission	Hospital transfer/admission
Prophylactic intravenous antibiotic timing	Prophylactic intravenous antibiotic timing	Prophylactic intravenous antibiotic timing
	Safe surgery checklist use	Safe surgery checklist use
	ASC facility volume data on selected ASC surgical procedures	ASC facility volume data on selected ASC surgical procedures
		Influenza vaccination coverage among health care personnel

Data from ASC safety. Available at: http://www.cms.gov/Medicare/Quality-Initiatives-Patient-Assessment-Instruments/ASC-Quality-Reporting. Accessed April 15, 2014.

health-related quality of life (HRQOL) following hand surgery.

To better capture HRQOL related to upper extremity function, several hand-specific measures exist. Two commonly used general measures of hand-related HRQOL are the Disabilities of the Arm, Shoulder and Hand (DASH) and the Michigan Hand Outcomes Questionnaire (MHQ). The DASH is a 30-item patient questionnaire that has been used for a variety of acute and chronic hand conditions among adults.[21] The DASH consists of 2 domains: upper extremity disability and symptoms, with additional optional modules relating to work and sports. An abbreviated version, the Quick DASH, has only 11 questions, and both versions can be adapted for touchpad administration. The MHQ is similar to DASH but is hand specific (does not include shoulder and elbow), and specifically assess both hands, adjusting for hand dominance.[22] Furthermore, the MHQ includes additional domains regarding hand appearance and patient satisfaction. A brief version of the MHQ has been developed and retains each of the original domains. Both the DASH and MHQ have been translated into many languages, and are widely used to assess outcomes after hand interventions following both acute and chronic hand conditions in adults.[23–26] To date, there are no validated instruments that capture hand-specific HRQOL among children.

Hand surgery cares for a diverse set of populations and problems. This heterogeneity limits the ability of measures such as the DASH and MHQ to capture the whole spectrum of improvements that may be meaningful to the patient.

For example, the DASH may be sensitive for a patient with disability related to posttraumatic wrist arthritis. However, the questions included on this instrument may not be appropriate for patients with virtually no upper extremity function, such as severe brachial plexus injuries or tetraplegia. One alternative to overcome the ceiling and floor effects of standardized surveys is to incorporate both qualitative and quantitative assessment, such as the Canadian Occupational Performance Measure (COPM). This measure is designed as a semistructured interview in which the patient identifies the 5 most important problems in daily functioning.[27] These problems are scored and then the patients' individual list of activities can be followed over time for meaningful changes. This client-centered technique is particularly helpful for severely disabled populations in which other measures are hampered by a floor effect (ie, the patient may improve functionally but this change is not reflected by a change in score). In this way, a person with tetraplegia is likely to have a high DASH score, indicating poor functioning, even following reconstruction. Using the COPM, the patient may identify independently holding a sandwich as an important goal and may reach this goal after reconstruction. The COPM would identify that improvement but the DASH score would likely remain unchanged, because of the constrained nature of the survey questions. The COPM has been used for a wide variety of problems and is a useful tool to assess a patient-centered view of quality of care.[28,29]

More recently the National Institutes of Health have introduced a new system for HRQOL measures, PROMIS (Patient-Reported Outcomes Measurement Information System). This program leverages modern psychometric techniques to standardize patient-reported outcome measures and provide a more efficient platform for administration.[30,31] At present, PROMIS measures HRQOL across physical, mental, and social health, and has been validated for many chronic conditions. In addition, item banks for adult and pediatric upper extremity functioning have been developed (**Table 2**). Groups, or banks, of generic items are used to capture each domain, and are ordered hierarchically using item-response theory (IRT) to minimize the overall number of questions required to capture a specific aspect of HRQOL. PROMIS also improves on the traditional paper/pencil administration formats by adapting item banks as computer adaptive tests (CATs). CATs are commonly used for standardized testing, such as the graduate management admission test and nursing board examinations, and facilitate the administration of IRT-based instruments by decreasing respondent burden without sacrificing the range of assessed abilities. Using CAT, the computer analyzes each answer, weights it, and then selects the most appropriate level of difficulty for follow-up questions.

This technique allows the most parsimonious survey to be given for each patient and significantly decreases the number of questions that

Table 2	
PROMIS adult self-reported health item banks	
Physical health	Upper extremity function Pain interference
Mental health	Anger Depression Anxiety Psychosocial illness impact
Social health	Ability to participate in social roles Satisfaction with social roles

must be answered, greatly reducing the time needed to take the survey. For example, among patients with foot and ankle disability, the general physical function test takes on average 47 seconds to complete.[32] This large National Institutes of Health endeavor with freely available instruments and ease of data storage and data analysis will redefine the way patient-reported outcomes will be measured in the future.

SATISFACTION

Recent events in health care reform have increasingly recognized patients as consumers, actively involved in their personal health care decisions as well as how health care is delivered in the United States.[33] Patient satisfaction with their outcomes and their experience is considered an essential metric of quality, and is empirically measured across hospitals. In 1995, the Agency for Healthcare Research and Quality (AHRQ) launched the Consumer Assessment of Healthcare Providers and Systems (CAHPS) program. This multiyear initiative is designed to assess and improve patient experiences within the health care system. Standardized surveys, such as the Hospital CAHPS (H-CAHPS), are given to patients to capture their personal perspectives on care. The H-CAHPS instrument contains 32 items that are compiled into 6 composite topics (nurse communication, physician communication, responsiveness of the hospital staff, pain management, communication regarding medications, and discharge information), 2 individual topics (cleanliness and quietness of the hospital environment), and 2 global topics (overall hospital rating, willingness to recommend hospital).[34] Patient experience is distinct from patient-reported outcomes, and focuses on the environment in which care was delivered, not the outcomes that the patient achieved, such as disability, disease-free recurrence, or the ability to return to work.

Although measures of patient experience have been met enthusiasm as an opportunity to improve care, several important limitations exist. First, the accuracy of the responses remains unclear. Patients often have difficulty remembering an experience because of delirium, sleep deprivation, pain, anxiety, and stress related to their condition requiring hospitalization, any of which could significantly influence their responses. For example, a CAHPS measure of patient-surgeon communication includes: "Before you left the surgical facility, did the surgeon discuss the outcome of your surgery with you?"[35] It is possible that a patient recovering from anesthesia may not remember talking to the surgeon, and rate the experience

lower based on this measure. In contrast, the quietness of the hospital environment is a metric captured on CAHPS instruments. Patients who are hospitalized in an intensive care setting, sedated, and unaware of their surroundings may not remember the noisiness of monitors and the bustle of the intensive care unit at night, and may rate their experience more favorably along this metric. Furthermore, it has been postulated that experience may not be correlated with hospital or surgeon performance, and may be irrelevant to quality.[36] However, CAHPS scores are correlated with other hospital quality metrics, indicating that they capture a distinct, but important, aspect of health care quality.[34] CAHPS scores have now been included in the CMS Hospital Compare program, and are publically available hospital metrics of performance, published and updated online. In addition, scores of patient experience are increasingly tied to financial incentives, underscoring their role in quality assessment and improvement in the health care system.

COST

Quality of care must be provided at a reasonable cost in order to efficiently use scarce health care resources and distribute services equitably across populations. Health care costs in the United States continue to accelerate rapidly. Compared with other developing countries, the United States spends 2.5 more on health care costs per capita, more than $8000 per person, with most being spent in the private sector.[37] Compare that with the health care systems in Japan, the United Kingdom, and Europe, where far less is spent, and not spent from the private sector. Although several causes have been cited for this, the increased expenditures in the United States are largely caused by increased service use, rather than other potential explanations such as price inflation.[38] Although explicit discussions of the costs of care when considering health care policy are sensitive, and often politically unfavorable, understanding the relative value of each dollar spent is essential to distribute scarce resources effectively.

Cost analyses, such as cost effective analysis or cost benefit analyses, can evaluate the financial burden of treatment options in the setting of potential benefits.[39,40] Benefits may include the absence of mortality, the decline of disability, and improvement in quality of life, and are often measured in units of benefit over time, such as quality-adjusted life years. Quality-of-life benefits can be assigned value by the use of utilities, which are valued on a scale of 0 for death and 1 equaling perfect health. Health utilities are calculated by asking respondents drawn from the general population how much healthy life they would give up or risk to have the theoretic medical condition cured.[41] The overall cost/ benefit ratio is calculated using a series of simulated exercises to generate an overall estimate. This type of methodology works well for chronic diseases associated with high morbidity, such as renal failure or heart failure. In these scenarios, the average respondent would willingly trade a significant length of life span in order to avoid dialysis.[42] However, trade-offs and outcomes in hand surgery are subtle and more difficult to measure.[43,44] For example, palmar fasciectomy for Dupuytren disease can greatly alleviate disabling finger contractures. However, mortality associated with this procedure is virtually nonexistent, and the concept of trading years of life for a straighter finger is much more difficult for a responder to conceptualize. Thus, many hand conditions get a very high utility value, or not much different than perfect health, which may skew an analysis to suggest that the costs outweigh the small benefits for hand conditions, and hand surgery may be deemed not to be cost-effective.[44] To date, the methods of simulating risks, benefits, and tradeoffs for safer procedures, such as hand surgery, remains limited. Future research that systematically quantifies empirical estimates of the outcomes most relevant in hand surgery, such as the ability to return to work, pain, and improved independence with activities of daily living, will allow more sensitive analyses that can better inform health care policy.

SUMMARY

Quality assessment and improvement in hand surgery remains underexplored. However, recent efforts in other surgical subspecialty fields, such as cardiac and orthopedic surgery, can inform early efforts to create benchmarks for surgical performance and clinical care that will increase the quality of care that will be provided in the future.

REFERENCES

1. Medicare compare website. Available at: https://data.medicare.gov/data/hospital-compare. Accessed March 14, 2014.
2. Chung KC, Shauver MJ. Measuring quality in health care and its implications for pay-for-performance initiatives. Hand Clin 2009;25:71–81, vii.
3. Kohn LT, Corrigan JM, Donaldson MS, editors. To err is human: building a safer health system. Washington, DC: National Academy Press, Institute of Medicine; 1999.
4. Russo A, Elixhauser A, Steiner C, et al. Hospital-based Ambulatory Surgery, 2007: Statistical Brief #86. Healthcare Cost and Utilization Project. Rockville (MD): Agency for Healthcare Policy and Research; 2010. PMID: 21452492.
5. Cullen KA, Hall MJ, Golosinskiy A. Ambulatory Surgery in the United States, 2006. National Health Stat Report 2009;28(11):1–25. PMID: 19294964.
6. Fecho K, Lunney AT, Boysen PG, et al. Postoperative mortality after inpatient surgery: incidence and risk factors. Ther Clin Risk Manag 2008;4:681–8.
7. Birkmeyer JD, Dimick JB. Understanding and reducing variation in surgical mortality. Annu Rev Med 2009;60:405–15.
8. Birkmeyer JD. Progress and challenges in improving surgical outcomes. Br J Surg 2012;99:1467–9.
9. Finks JF, Kole KL, Yenumula PR, et al. Predicting risk for serious complications with bariatric surgery: results from the Michigan Bariatric Surgery Collaborative. Ann Surg 2011;254:633–40.
10. Goodney PP, Siewers AE, Stukel TA, et al. Is surgery getting safer? National trends in operative mortality. J Am Coll Surg 2002;195:219–27.
11. Daley J, Khuri SF, Henderson W, et al. Risk adjustment of the postoperative morbidity rate for the comparative assessment of the quality of surgical care: results of the National Veterans Affairs Surgical Risk Study. J Am Coll Surg 1997;185:328–40.
12. Khuri SF, Henderson WG, Daley J, et al. Successful implementation of the Department of Veterans Affairs' National Surgical Quality Improvement Program in the private sector: the Patient Safety in Surgery study. Ann Surg 2008;248:329–36.
13. Khuri SF, Daley J, Henderson W, et al. Risk adjustment of the postoperative mortality rate for the comparative assessment of the quality of surgical care: results of the National Veterans Affairs Surgical Risk Study. J Am Coll Surg 1997;185:315–27.
14. Khuri SF, Daley J, Henderson W, et al. The Department of Veterans Affairs' NSQIP: the first national, validated, outcome-based, risk-adjusted, and peer-controlled program for the measurement and enhancement of the quality of surgical care. National VA Surgical Quality Improvement Program. Ann Surg 1998;228:491–507.
15. Hall BL, Hamilton BH, Richards K, et al. Does surgical quality improve in the American College of Surgeons National Surgical Quality Improvement Program: an evaluation of all participating hospitals. Ann Surg 2009;250:363–76.
16. Campbell DA Jr, Henderson WG, Englesbe MJ, et al. Surgical site infection prevention: the importance of operative duration and blood transfusion–results of the first American College of Surgeons-National Surgical Quality Improvement Program Best Practices Initiative. J Am Coll Surg 2008;207:810–20.

17. Fischer JP, Nelson JA, Kovach SJ, et al. Impact of obesity on outcomes in breast reconstruction: analysis of 15,937 patients from the ACS-NSQIP datasets. J Am Coll Surg 2013;217(4):656–64.

18. Mathis MR, Naughton NN, Shanks AM, et al. Patient selection for day case-eligible surgery: identifying those at high risk for major complications. Anesthesiology 2013;119(6):1310–21.

19. ASC safety. Available at: http://www.cms.gov/Medicare/Quality-Initiatives-Patient-Assessment-Instruments/ASC-Quality-Reporting. Accessed April 15, 2014.

20. Klum M, Wolf MB, Hahn P, et al. Normative data on wrist function. J Hand Surg Am 2012;37(10):2050–60.

21. DASH home page. Available at: http://www.dash.iwh.on.ca/. Accessed March 12, 2014.

22. MHQ home page. Available at: http://sitemaker.umich.edu/mhq/overview. Accessed March 14, 2014.

23. Karantana A, Downing ND, Forward DP, et al. Surgical treatment of distal radial fractures with a volar locking plate versus conventional percutaneous methods: a randomized controlled trial. J Bone Joint Surg Am 2013;95(19):1737–44.

24. Trumble TE, Vedder NB, Seiler JG 3rd, et al. Zone-II flexor tendon repair: a randomized prospective trial of active place-and-hold therapy compared with passive motion therapy. J Bone Joint Surg Am 2010;92(6):1381–9.

25. Chung KC, Burns PB, Wilgis EF, et al. A multicenter clinical trial in rheumatoid arthritis comparing silicone metacarpophalangeal joint arthroplasty with medical treatment. J Hand Surg Am 2009;34(5):815–23.

26. Umraw N, Chan Y, Gomez M, et al. Effective hand function assessment after burn injuries. J Burn Care Rehabil 2004;25(1):134–9.

27. Law M, Baptiste S, McColl M, et al. The Canadian occupational performance measure: an outcome measure for occupational therapy. Can J Occup Ther 1990;57(2):82–7.

28. Wangdell J, Fridén J. Satisfaction and performance in patient selected goals after grip reconstruction in tetraplegia. J Hand Surg Eur Vol 2010;35(7):563–8.

29. Wijk U, Wollmark M, Kopylov P, Tägil M. Outcomes of proximal interphalangeal joint pyrocarbon implants. J Hand Surg Am 2010;35(1):38–43.

30. PROMIS history. Available at: http://www.nihpromis.org/Documents/PROMIS_The_First_Four_Years.pdf. Accessed March 14, 2014.

31. Cella D, Yount S, Rothrock N, et al, on behalf of the PROMIS Cooperative Group. The Patient Reported Outcomes Measurement Information System (PROMIS): progress of an NIH Roadmap Cooperative Group during its first two years. Med Care 2007;45(5):S3–11.

32. Hung M, Baumhauer JF, Latt LD, et al. Validation of PROMIS® Physical Function computerized adaptive tests for orthopaedic foot and ankle outcome research. National Orthopaedic Foot & Ankle Outcomes Research Network. Clin Orthop Relat Res 2013;471(11):3466–74.

33. Jayadevappa R, Chhatre S. Patient centered care - a conceptual model and review of the state of the art. Open Health Serv Policy J 2011;4:15–25.

34. Jha AK, Orav EJ, Zheng J, et al. Patients' perception of hospital care in the United States. N Engl J Med 2008;359:1921–31.

35. CAHPS surgical survey. Available at: http://www.facs.org/ahp/cahps/reporting-measures.pdf. Accessed March 14, 2014.

36. Lyu H, Wick EC, Housman M, et al. Patient satisfaction as a possible indicator of quality surgical care. JAMA Surg 2013;148(4):362–7.

37. Organization for Economic Cooperation and Development. Health Data. 2012. Available at: http://www.oecd.org. Accessed April 15, 2014.

38. Fisher ES, Bynum JP, Skinner JS. Slowing the growth of health care costs–lessons from regional variation. N Engl J Med 2009;360:849–52.

39. Song JW, Chung KC, Prosser LA. Treatment of ulnar neuropathy at the elbow: cost-utility analysis. J Hand Surg Am 2012;37(8):1617–29.

40. Thoma A, Wong VH, Sprague S, et al. A cost-utility analysis of open and endoscopic carpal tunnel release. Can J Plast Surg 2006;14(1):15–20.

41. CEA registry. Available at: https://research.tufts-nemc.org/cear4/Home.aspx. Accessed March 14, 2014.

42. Smith D, Loewenstein G, Jepson C, et al. Mispredicting and misremembering: patients with renal failure overestimate improvements in quality of life after a kidney transplant. Health Psychol 2008;27:653–8.

43. Chen NC, Shauver MJ, Chung KC. A primer on use of decision analysis methodology in hand surgery. J Hand Surg Am 2009;34:983–90.

44. Chen NC, Shauver MJ, Chung KC. Cost-effectiveness of open partial fasciectomy, needle aponeurotomy, and collagenase injection for Dupuytren contracture. J Hand Surg Am 2011;36:1826–34.e32.

Collaborative Quality Improvement in Surgery

Jennifer F. Waljee, MD, MS, MPH[a,*], Nancy J.O. Birkmeyer, PhD[b,c]

KEYWORDS

- Quality collaborative • Regional collaborative • Quality of care • Surgery

KEY POINTS

- Collaborative quality assessment and improvement models have emerged as a novel and effective strategy for examining practice patterns and outcomes in surgery.
- Unlike pay-for-performance programs, pay-for-participation programs do not incentivize or punish participants based on outcomes but focus on the collection of high-quality, rigorous, detailed clinical data that are then provided in an aggregate format for feedback to stakeholders.
- Quality collaboratives in surgery have resulted in improved perioperative outcomes by lowering perioperative complication rates, unplanned readmissions, and surgery-associated health care costs.

QUALITY OF CARE IN THE UNITED STATES

It is well documented that there is wide variation in surgical care in the United States.[1,2] Differences in outcomes can occur for several reasons, such as random variation or differences in baseline risk. However, variation often signals important discrepancies in surgical quality, highlighting opportunities to improve the efficiency, effectiveness, and safety of surgery.[2]

Millions of Americans undergo surgery each year in the United States, with expenditures exceeding $500 billion and accounting for approximately 40% of national health care spending.[3–5] Preventable perioperative complications result in substantial disability, longer hospital stays, and dramatically increased health care expenditures. For example, the occurrence of a single postoperative complication, such as pneumonia, dramatically increases the cost of care nearly 10-fold.[6–8] These expenses result in diminished hospital reimbursement and lower profit margins and are primarily borne by large third-party payers.[9]

In this context, professional societies and payers are keen on identifying the most effective strategies to improve the safety and efficiency of surgical care. This review highlights the development and features of collaborative quality improvement programs, their advantages and examples of successful collaborations for several surgical conditions, and their potential application for surgeons caring for patients with upper extremity trauma and disability.

STRATEGIES TO IMPROVE SURGICAL QUALITY

Given the relationship between variation in quality and accelerating health care expenditures, recent health care policy has increasingly focused on strategies that achieve high-quality care while efficiently using scarce health care resources. Previous efforts

Disclosures: None.
[a] Section of Plastic Surgery, Department of Surgery, University of Michigan Medical Center, University of Michigan Health System, 1500 East Medical Center Drive, 2131 Taubman Center, Ann Arbor, MI 48109, USA; [b] Michigan Bariatric Surgery Collaborative, Center for Healthcare Outcomes and Policy, North Campus Research Complex, 2800 Plymouth Road, B016, Ann Arbor, MI 48109, USA; [c] Department of Surgery, University of Michigan Medical Center, 1500 East Medial Center Drive, Ann Arbor, MI 48109, USA
* Corresponding author.
E-mail address: filip@umich.edu

have included public reporting of outcomes, regionalization of care into centers of excellence, pay-for-performance strategies, and, in recent years, collaborative quality improvement. For example, in 2008, the World Health Organization created a checklist of perioperative safety measures. These instruments can be reviewed by individuals perioperatively to ensure that best practices are being followed, or at least considered.[10–12] Although the use of safety checklists is associated with measurable declines in perioperative complications and morbidity, a causal relationship between checklists and improvement in quality remains unclear. It is possible that implementing safety checklists increases the awareness of performance among the entire team, rather than due to any specific elements of the checklist itself. Furthermore, their effectiveness relies on their ability to be implemented, which may wane over time.[13]

Other strategies have focused on increasing the transparency and accessibility of quality measures. For example, the Centers for Medicare and Medicaid Services (CMS) routinely release data regarding hospital performance through the web-based Hospital Compare program.[14] Although publically reporting quality measures has strong face validity, and is increasingly popular, these strategies are not clearly linked with improved quality or selective referral to higher performing centers. Furthermore, the accuracy and validity of publically reported measures remains uncertain.[15] Most patients choose providers because of local or regional logistical factors, and many have difficulty interpreting quality measures and placing these into appropriate context.[16–19]

Finally, large payers have proposed financial incentives for providers who achieve superior compliance. For example, reimbursement for care has been linked with specific processes of care, such as perioperative antibiotic prophylaxis as proposed through the Surgical Care Improvement Project.[20] More recently, the Affordable Care Act directed the CMS to penalize those hospitals with higher 30-day readmission rates for common conditions.[21] Although this approach is appealing, compliance with quality measures is not correlated with improved outcomes after surgery, and this clearly suggests that more is needed to improve quality on a population-based level.[22–24]

COLLABORATIVE QUALITY IMPROVEMENT

In contrast to pay-for-performance models, pay-for-participation quality assessment and improvement strategies have evolved (**Table 1**). In this cooperative approach, large payers provide financial support and infrastructure to establish collaborations among hospitals and health care centers that are directed at improving the quality of care for patients with a specific condition or undergoing a specific type of surgical procedure.[25] In this context, large payers include those insurers and

Table 1
Characteristics of pay for performance versus pay for participation quality assessment and improvement models

	Pay for Performance	Pay for Participation
Strategy	Reimbursement directly linked specific metrics (compliance with best practices, achievement of superior outcomes)	Financial incentives are linked to provider participation in cooperative quality assessment groups (eg, accurate, timely submission of clinical data)
Example	CMS penalties for hospitals with worse than expected 30-d readmission outcomes	MSQC: statewide consortium of hospitals performing general and vascular surgical procedures in Michigan, funded by BCBSM/BCN
Advantages	Tangible financial rewards Directly addresses cost implications of poor quality care	Regular feedback of clinical data Access to a network of providers with common goals/interests
Drawbacks	Limited data to support a clear link between many processes of care and quality improvement Outcomes that are appropriately adjusted for risk and reliability are rarely available Potential for gaming the system	Labor intensive to organize and maintain Challenging to overcome culture of competition in the health care marketplace

Abbreviations: BCBSM/BCN, Blue Cross Blue Shield of Michigan/Blue Care Network; MSQC, Michigan Surgical Quality Collaborative.

employers who directly or indirectly finance health care.[26] Although many quality collaboratives are funded by large payers, others, such as the Northern New England Cardiovascular Disease Study group, are supported by participating hospitals, and participation of large payers is not inherent in the structure of these organizations.

Quality collaboratives are often, but not always, grouped naturally by region. **Fig. 1** depicts a conceptual model of quality collaborative improvement in health care. In the collaborative, each hospital or site collects longitudinal, prospective clinical data regarding patient characteristics, clinical outcomes, and relevant processes of care, which are then submitted to a coordinating center. Data are obtained at regular intervals from the medical record by trained chart abstractors using standardized definitions and maintained in a large clinical registry. Registries include detailed patient clinical and sociodemographic information including risk factors, processes of care, and outcomes. For example, the Michigan Society of Thoracic and Cardiovascular Surgeons (MSTCVS) uses an infrastructure developed by the Society of Thoracic Surgeons (STS) to detail relevant clinical events (eg, complications, mortality) after standard cardiac surgical procedures such as coronary artery bypass grafting.

Hospitals and surgeons receive regular feedback regarding their performance at timed intervals from the coordinating center. Participants convene at regular intervals, such as biannually or quarterly, to review the data and interpret areas of improvement, concern, or variation. Changes in practices and resultant outcomes can be tracked, and the most successful strategies, or best practices, can be implemented in a standard manner. Participation in the collaborative is voluntary, but compensation is provided for those centers that maintain data and participation standards. Hospitals and physician groups are compensated for their participation and data collection efforts, regardless of their individual performance or how they rank compared with other hospitals.

CRITICAL ELEMENTS OF A QUALITY COLLABORATIVE

In essence, quality collaboratives are groups of hospitals and physicians who come together to exchange data for the purpose of improving care.[27] One of the first examples of quality collaborative improvement is the Northern New England Cardiovascular Disease Study Group.[28] Established in 1987, this consortium includes cardiothoracic surgeons, interventional cardiologists, nurses, anesthesiologists, perfusionists, administrators, and scientists from 8 centers across Maine, New Hampshire, and Vermont and has collected data from over 190,000 procedures over 24 years. Since that time, quality collaborative models have continued to evolve and expand throughout the United States. Although each has unique characteristics, quality collaboratives all share 4 critical elements: rigorous data, timely feedback, transparent reporting, and collaborative improvement (**Table 2**).

The cornerstone of any quality collaborative is accurate and reliable data. Data should be procedure specific (laparoscopic gastric banding vs Roux-en-Y gastric bypass) as well as detail all relevant clinical outcomes (complication rates, readmission rates, length of stay, mortality). Furthermore, registries must contain specific information regarding patient sociodemographic characteristics and clinical risk factors in order to adequately risk adjust or account for the baseline differences in risk that may influence patient outcomes. Finally, registries should contain the processes of care that are relevant

Performance standards	Performance measurement
Identify relevant measures	Develop data management system
Set goals and targets	Systematic data collection
Communicate expectations	Continually refine indicators and measures

Collaborative quality improvement

Progress reporting	Quality improvement process
Risk and reliability-adjusted data analysis	Use data to revise and improve practice
Routine dissemination to stakeholders	Create learning organization
Maintain data privacy standards	Multidisciplinary implementation

Fig. 1. Conceptual model of collaborative quality improvement. (*Adapted from* Public Health Foundation. Turning point: performance management project and publications. Available at: http://www.phf.org/resourcestools/pages/turning_point_project_publications.aspx. Accessed May 7, 2014.)

Table 2
Key elements of collaborative quality improvement

Element	Relevance	Example
Rigorous data	Accurate and reliable data provides the foundation on which performance can be assessed and improvement strategies developed Outcomes data should be appropriately adjusted for differences in baseline risk, as well as for reliability to account for the heterogeneity of sample sizes in a quality collaborative	Postoperative complication events (eg, anastomotic leak after bariatric surgery), adjusted for common patient risk factors
Timely feedback	Performance data is provided at regular intervals to provide information regarding recent practice patterns and to promote continuous improvement	Quarterly meetings between program directors, surgeons, and hospital leadership to review individual and aggregate data
Data protection	Individual surgeon and hospital data should be provided as appropriate for self-review Data presentation on a larger scale should include aggregate or deidentified data to protect participants	Postoperative readmission rates are presented in aggregate to stakeholders
Collective improvement	A multidisciplinary approach to developing quality improvement strategies is optimal in order to leverage the expertise of all participants (eg, nursing staff, physicians, patient advocates)	Nursing-driven documentation of the use of intracranial monitoring of patients who have experienced trauma

to the condition or surgical procedure of interest (such as the use of perioperative antibiotics or β-blockers).

In addition to rigorous data, timely feedback of data is provided to participants at regular intervals. Typically, this occurs at regularly scheduled meetings between providers, surgeons, and program coordinators in which performance data are reviewed. Risk-adjusted outcomes are then reported to participants. Regression-based time series analyses are used to determine longitudinal trends in care, adjusting for measurable changes in patient characteristics over time. Data can then be compared over time, to hospital and regional averages, and against national trends. Data can also be linked to specific processes or interventions that have been implemented to improve outcomes in order to examine effectiveness.

In addition, performance data should be provided in a transparent manner that is easy to interpret and is provided either in a confidential manner to individual surgeons or in a deidentified format when presented in a group format (**Fig. 2**). Reports can then be used by hospitals to compare their own performance against other systems, or against aggregate means. Payers require regular reporting from participants to ensure data quality and have access to data in order to follow variation in care.

Finally, collaboratives work together to interpret data, determine needs and strategies for improvement, and ensure that the interests of the group are being met.[25] For example, an analysis from the Michigan Bariatric Surgery Collaborative (MBSC) revealed wide variation in the use of inferior vena cava (IVC) filters for prevention of postoperative pulmonary embolism. Further investigation revealed that IVC filters were associated with significant risk and yielded no protective effect from pulmonary embolism.[29] After dissemination of this information across the collaborative, the use of IVC filters, and their associated complications, dropped dramatically in subsequent years.[9]

QUALITY COLLABORATIVES IN PRACTICE: THE MICHIGAN EXPERIENCE

In Michigan, the Blue Cross Blue Shield of Michigan and Blue Care Network (BCBSM/BCN) and surgical leaders within the state have developed several regional collaboratives for common surgical conditions and procedures, which are detailed below.[9,25] To date, most collaboratives have focused on common conditions that are associated with high costs per episode, such as cardiovascular disease. However, these have widely expanded in recent years to now include breast disease, bariatric surgery,

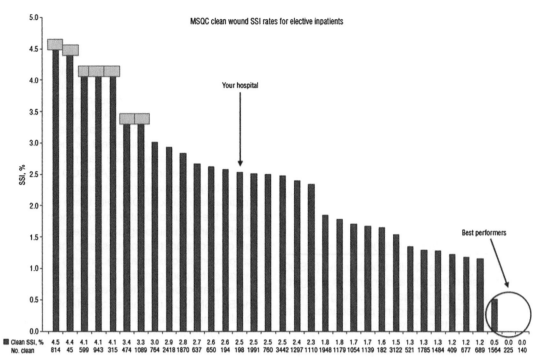

Fig. 2. An example of clinical data (eg, surgical site infection [SSI] rates) provided through quality collaborative improvement programs. (*From* Campbell DA, Englesbe MJ, Kubus JJ, et al. Accelerating the pace of surgical quality improvement. The power of hospital collaboration. Arch Surg 2010;145(10):986; with permission.)

urologic conditions, spine surgery, and trauma. The following discussion highlights specific examples of these collaboratives in practice in Michigan.

Cardiac Surgery

In Michigan, one of the oldest efforts to bring surgeons, hospitals, and payers together in a cooperative approach is through the MSTCVS. The MSTCVS was founded in 1965, when 17 thoracic surgeons came together for the purpose of reviewing cases and current practices in the context of scientific evidence. This effort was expanded in subsequent years to include a prospective clinical registry, and is now funded by BCBSM/ BCN to create a voluntary consortium.[30] Data are collected through a national platform developed by the STS and obtained using nurses trained in chart abstraction. Given the variability in billing practices, participants are given hypothetical case scenarios, and responses are reviewed among all participants to improve consistency. Site visits are conducted on a routine basis by collaborative staff, and data are audited regularly to ensure completeness and accuracy.

The MSTCVS rates hospital performance using an 11-item composite measure of quality that incorporates risk-adjusted mortality, complications, and technical aspects of care.[9] Using this metric, participating hospitals have improved performance

compared with national averages and are within the 10th percentile nationwide. In addition to improved outcomes, this collaborative has leveraged its data to identify best practices, such as blood conservation and internal mammary use.[31,32] In this way, the Michigan experience has served as a template for collaborative quality improvement in cardiac surgery going forward.[33]

Bariatric Surgery

The MBSC was established in 2006 and currently collects data on over 5000 patients each year, nearly 95% of all patients who undergo bariatric surgery, from 40 hospitals across the state performing bariatric surgery. Coordinated at the University of Michigan, this collaborative has established a longitudinal registry of patients undergoing bariatric surgery, specifically collecting data regarding patient preoperative risk factors, surgery received, and perioperative care. In addition, the registry routinely collects data regarding self-reported measures including clinical outcomes, such as weight loss, resolution of comorbid conditions, postoperative complications, and mortality. Patient-reported outcomes are also collected, such as disability and patient satisfaction.

As with the MSTCVS, the MBSC is funded by BCBSM/BCN, the largest third-party payer in Michigan. From this effort, annual complications have declined among participating hospitals. Overall complication rates have declined from 8.7% to 6.6% between 2007 and 2009 and greater improvement has been demonstrated compared with the national average.[9] In addition to improving postoperative mortality, data available from the MBSC registry have been used to identify patients at risk for major complications from bariatric surgery and understand the interplay between surgeon skill and postoperative complications.[34,35] Finally, data from the MBSC have been used to better understand the risks and benefits of common perioperative practices, such as prevention of venous thromboembolism.[29,36,37]

General and Vascular Surgery

The Michigan Surgical Quality Collaborative (MSQC) was established in 2005 and maintains a registry of 66 hospitals in Michigan performing common general and vascular surgery procedures.[38] The MSQC uses a platform developed by the American College of Surgeons National Surgical Quality Improvement Program (ACS-NSQIP) to maintain a detailed registry of patient clinical and sociodemographic information, perioperative processes of care and events, and clinical outcomes.[39–41] The collaborative maintains the pay-for-participation approach as described earlier, and is financially supported by the BCBSM/BCN. Providers and program leaders meet quarterly to discuss aggregate results and identify potential quality improvement strategies.

As seen among hospitals participating in the MBSC, participation in MSQC has resulted in significant declines in morbidity for common inpatient surgical procedures.[39] Data available from the quality collaborative have also been used to provide a closer view of the differences in clinical and cost outcomes among vulnerable patient groups, such as the frail or elderly. In addition, data can be linked to existing quality metrics, such as the Hospital Consumer Assessment of Healthcare Providers and Surveys program, to provide deeper insight into provider performance.[42] Finally, quality collaborative data can be leveraged for population-based comparative effectiveness analyses of common perioperative processes of care. For example, the evidence supporting use of bowel preparation for colectomy has long been disputed because of heterogeneous data primarily drawn from single-center studies. Recently, however, data from the MSQC have demonstrated that bowel preparation before colectomy is associated with decreased rates of surgical site infections, providing rigorous, population-based evidence to support a change in surgical practice.[43]

Trauma Surgery

A continuous, systematic approach to improving care for patients who have experienced trauma has been endorsed as an optimal strategy by leading professional organizations.[44–46] Current efforts have combined established benchmarks and quality metrics with the existing platform developed by NSQIP to create a collaborative approach to quality improvement and measurement for the care of patients who have experienced trauma. In 2006, the ACS Committee on Trauma (ACS-COT) combined an existing nationwide trauma registry, the National Trauma Data Bank (NTDB), with these resources to create the Trauma Quality Improvement Program (TQIP). Through this program, surgeons and hospitals can compare their processes of care and clinical outcomes to external benchmarks and national averages for peer centers. These efforts have been disseminated on a statewide level, and in 2009, the BCBSM/BCN formalized the Michigan Trauma Quality Improvement Project.

Consolidating data in national registries has allowed for the critical analysis of common practices in trauma surgery, and the implementation of continuous quality assessment and improvement through TQIP yields better outcomes.[47,48] Population-based data derived from TQIP can highlight the variation in evidence-based practice. For example, the use of intracranial pressure monitoring for patients who have experienced trauma and are severely injured varies widely, despite existing guidelines supporting its use as the standard of care. Finally, population-based data can be used to provide more reliable estimates of outcomes among patients who have traumatic injuries, which can be used to streamline resources to at-risk patients.[49]

ADVANTAGES OF QUALITY COLLABORATIVE IMPROVEMENT

From the examples outlined above, it is clear that collaborative quality improvement offers substantial return on investment. Results from the Michigan experience suggest that hospitals that participate in regional collaborative improvement programs experience gains in quality much faster than hospitals that do not participate. The large sample sizes and associated statistical power allow for robust estimates of the potential association between changes in processes of care and patient outcomes. Furthermore, streamlined data registries offer rapid feedback on outcomes. Declining perioperative morbidity among participants translates to substantial cost savings, specifically for large payers.[9,50] However, the benefits are not just financial. Quality collaboratives gather detailed clinical data on a population-based level, which is often far superior to that collected in claims or administrative data. For example, the MBSC is one of the few quality collaboratives that collected population-based patient-reported outcomes, such as self-reported disability and patient satisfaction. Although the purpose of quality collaboratives is to improve quality of care, they provide a unique laboratory for population-based research and set up a natural experiment for quality improvement efforts.[51] In this way, quality collaboratives represent an ideal opportunity for population-based comparative effectiveness research.

In addition to these empirical measures, there are other, less tangible benefits of collaborative quality improvement. Quality collaboratives represent an opportunity to share best practices and common interests across systems in a noncompetitive or adversarial way. Quality collaboratives also provide a network of providers that can support one another and identify successful strategies for navigating the changing landscape of health care delivery. Finally, participants may develop a heightened awareness of safety culture and may be more cognizant of their practice patterns and the need for critically assessing the clinical decisions on a continuous basis.[26,52]

CHALLENGES OF QUALITY COLLABORATIVES

Despite these successes, collaborative efforts to improve quality have important limitations. First, organizing partnerships across hospitals is logistically difficult and labor intensive, despite generous financial support from large payers. Collaboratives require the assembly of a large, committed team with expertise in health care quality, health service delivery, epidemiology, complex data management, and statistical analysis. Amassing the resources necessary for this endeavor is difficult and expensive. There are often few direct financial incentives to participate in collaboratives, and large payers bear the cost of the data infrastructure and the processes of the collaborative. The benefits and rewards from participation are not immediate, and cost savings because of shorter length of stays, fewer complications, and improved care are seen over time, rather than immediately. Furthermore, for those lower-risk conditions in which outcomes such as disability and diminished health-related quality of life are more common than mortality or readmission, payers may be less enthusiastic about participating collaborative improvement. For these conditions, such as hernia repair or carpal tunnel surgery, the health benefits are much more difficult to define and the potential

for cost reduction is less clear. Finally, surgeons may be reticent to release data regarding negative outcomes or poor compliance to standards of care. Quality collaboratives require that hospitals and surgeons set aside competing interests, which is difficult in a financially risky health care market. Providers may also fear that data could be linked to reimbursement or publically reported, increasing reluctance to participate. Nonetheless, the previous successes in collaborative quality improvement indicate that it is effective in promoting high-value health care and will likely to be the standard going forward.

FUTURE DIRECTIONS IN QUALITY COLLABORATIVE IMPROVEMENT

In conclusion, collaborative quality improvement has demonstrated success in improving quality and reducing health care costs in several state-based examples. In the future, the integration of patient-reported outcomes, postacute health care use, and employment/vocational burden into quality collaborative initiatives will create an opportunity to apply these models to other conditions, such as upper extremity disability, which are relatively lower risk, but have a profound, lasting effect on disability and health-related quality of life.

REFERENCES

1. Birkmeyer JD, Siewers AE, Finlayson EV, et al. Hospital volume and surgical mortality in the United States. N Engl J Med 2002;346:1128–37.
2. Birkmeyer JD, Dimick JB. Understanding and reducing variation in surgical mortality. Annu Rev Med 2009;60:405–15.
3. Russo A, Elixhauser A, Steiner C, et al. Healthcare Cost and Utilization Project Statistical Briefs (Brief #86). Rockville (MD): Agency for Health Care Policy and Research; 2010.
4. Cullen KA, Hall MJ, Golosinskiy A. Ambulatory Surgery in the United States, 2006. National Center for Health Statistics 2009;28(11):1–25.
5. Fecho K, Lunney AT, Boysen PG, et al. Postoperative mortality after inpatient surgery: incidence and risk factors. Ther Clin Risk Manag 2008;4:681–8.
6. Englesbe MJ, Dimick J, Mathur A, et al. Who pays for biliary complications following liver transplant? A business case for quality improvement. Am J Transplant 2006;6:2978–82.
7. Dimick JB, Weeks WB, Karia RJ, et al. Who pays for poor surgical quality? Building a business case for quality improvement. J Am Coll Surg 2006;202:933–7.
8. Dimick JB, Chen SL, Taheri PA, et al. Hospital costs associated with surgical complications: a report from the private-sector National Surgical Quality

Improvement Program. J Am Coll Surg 2004;199: 531–7.

9. Share DA, Campbell DA, Birkmeyer N, et al. How a regional collaborative of hospitals and physicians in Michigan cut costs and improved the quality of care. Health Aff (Millwood) 2011;30:636–45.

10. Haynes AB, Weiser TG, Berry WR, et al. A surgical safety checklist to reduce morbidity and mortality in a global population. N Engl J Med 2009;360: 491–9.

11. Abdel-Galil K. The WHO surgical safety checklist: are we measuring up? Br J Oral Maxillofac Surg 2010;48:397–8.

12. Birkmeyer JD. Strategies for improving surgical quality–checklists and beyond. N Engl J Med 2010;363:1963–5.

13. Birkmeyer JD. Progress and challenges in improving surgical outcomes. Br J Surg 2012;99:1467–9.

14. Werner RM, Bradlow ET. Relationship between Medicare's hospital compare performance measures and mortality rates. JAMA 2006;296:2694–702.

15. Dahlke AR, Chung JW, Holl JL, et al. Evaluation of initial participation in public reporting of American College of Surgeons NSQIP surgical outcomes on Medicare's Hospital Compare website. J Am Coll Surg 2014;218:374–80, 380.e1–5.

16. Finlayson SR, Birkmeyer JD, Tosteson AN, et al. Patient preferences for location of care: implications for regionalization. Med Care 1999;37:204–9.

17. Schwartz LM, Woloshin S, Welch HG. Can patients interpret health information? An assessment of the medical data interpretation test. Med Decis Making 2005;25:290–300.

18. Schwartz LM, Woloshin S, Welch HG. Risk communication in clinical practice: putting cancer in context. J Natl Cancer Inst Monogr 1999;(25):124–33.

19. Schwartz LM, Woloshin S, Birkmeyer JD. How do elderly patients decide where to go for major surgery? Telephone interview survey. BMJ 2005; 331:821.

20. Werner RM, Bradlow ET. Public reporting on hospital process improvements is linked to better patient outcomes. Health Aff (Millwood) 2010;29:1319–24.

21. Joynt KE, Jha AK. Thirty-day readmissions–truth and consequences. N Engl J Med 2012;366: 1366–9.

22. Nicholas LH, Osborne NH, Birkmeyer JD, et al. Hospital process compliance and surgical outcomes in medicare beneficiaries. Arch Surg 2010;145: 999–1004.

23. Hawn MT, Vick CC, Richman J, et al. Surgical site infection prevention: time to move beyond the surgical care improvement program. Ann Surg 2011; 254:494–9 [discussion: 499–501].

24. Shih T, Nicholas LH, Thumma JR, et al. Does pay-for-performance improve surgical outcomes? An evaluation of phase 2 of the premier hospital quality incentive demonstration. Ann Surg 2014; 259:677–81.

25. Birkmeyer NJ, Share D, Campbell DA Jr, et al. Partnering with payers to improve surgical quality: the Michigan plan. Surgery 2005;138:815–20.

26. Birkmeyer NJ, Birkmeyer JD. Strategies for improving surgical quality–should payers reward excellence or effort? N Engl J Med 2006;354: 864–70.

27. Foundation PH. From silos to systems. Using performance management to improve the public's heath. Performance Management National Excellence Collaborative; 2003. Available at: http://www.phf.org/resourcestools/Documents/silossystems.pdf. Accessed June 23, 2014.

28. O'Connor GT, Plume SK, Olmstead EM, et al. A regional intervention to improve the hospital mortality associated with coronary artery bypass graft surgery. The Northern New England Cardiovascular Disease Study Group. JAMA 1996;275: 841–6.

29. Birkmeyer NJ, Finks JF, English WJ, et al. Risks and benefits of prophylactic inferior vena cava filters in patients undergoing bariatric surgery. J Hosp Med 2013;8:173–7.

30. Prager RL, Armenti FR, Bassett JS, et al. Cardiac surgeons and the quality movement: the Michigan experience. Semin Thorac Cardiovasc Surg 2009; 21:20–7.

31. Paone G, Likosky DS, Brewer R, et al. Transfusion of 1 and 2 units of red blood cells is associated with increased morbidity and mortality. Ann Thorac Surg 2014;97:87–93 [discussion: 93–4].

32. Johnson SH, Theurer PF, Bell GF, et al. A statewide quality collaborative for process improvement: internal mammary artery utilization. Ann Thorac Surg 2010;90:1158–64 [discussion: 1164].

33. Speir AM, Rich JB, Crosby I, et al. Regional collaboration as a model for fostering accountability and transforming health care. Semin Thorac Cardiovasc Surg 2009;21:12–9.

34. Birkmeyer JD, Finks JF, O'Reilly A, et al. Surgical skill and complication rates after bariatric surgery. N Engl J Med 2013;369:1434–42.

35. Finks JF, Kole KL, Yenumula PR, et al. Predicting risk for serious complications with bariatric surgery: results from the Michigan Bariatric Surgery Collaborative. Ann Surg 2011;254:633–40.

36. Birkmeyer NJ, Finks JF, Carlin AM, et al. Comparative effectiveness of unfractionated and low-molecular-weight heparin for prevention of venous thromboembolism following bariatric surgery. Arch Surg 2012; 147:994–8.

37. Finks JF, English WJ, Carlin AM, et al. Predicting risk for venous thromboembolism with bariatric surgery: results from the Michigan Bariatric Surgery Collaborative. Ann Surg 2012;255:1100–4.

38. Campbell DA Jr, Kubus JJ, Henke PK, et al. The Michigan Surgical Quality Collaborative: a legacy of Shukri Khuri. Am J Surg 2009;198: S49–55.

39. Campbell DA Jr, Englesbe MJ, Kubus JJ, et al. Accelerating the pace of surgical quality improvement: the power of hospital collaboration. Arch Surg 2010;145: 985–91.

40. Sheetz KH, Guy K, Allison JH, et al. Improving the care of elderly adults undergoing surgery in Michigan. J Am Geriatr Soc 2014;62:352–7.

41. Sheetz KH, Waits SA, Terjimanian MN, et al. Cost of major surgery in the sarcopenic patient. J Am Coll Surg 2013;217:813–8.

42. Sheetz KH, Waits SA, Girotti ME, et al. Patients' perspectives of care and surgical outcomes in Michigan: an analysis using the CAHPS hospital survey. Ann Surg 2014;260(1):5–9.

43. Kim EK, Sheetz KH, Bonn J, et al. A statewide colectomy experience: the role of full bowel preparation in preventing surgical site infection. Ann Surg 2014;259:310–4.

44. Shafi S, Nathens AB, Cryer HG, et al. The trauma quality improvement program of the American College of Surgeons Committee on Trauma. J Am Coll Surg 2009;209:521–30.e1.

45. Hemmila MR, Jakubus JL, Wahl WL, et al. Detecting the blind spot: complications in the trauma registry and trauma quality improvement. Surgery 2007;142:439–48 [discussion: 448–9].

46. Crandall M, Zarzaur B, Tinkoff G. American Association for the Surgery of Trauma Prevention Committee topical overview: National Trauma Data Bank, geographic information systems, and teaching injury prevention. Am J Surg 2013;206:709–13.

47. Sarkar B, Brunsvold ME, Cherry-Bukoweic JR, et al. American College of Surgeons' Committee on Trauma Performance Improvement and Patient Safety program: maximal impact in a mature trauma center. J Trauma 2011;71:1447–53 [discussion: 1453–4].

48. Nathens AB, Cryer HG, Fildes J. The American College of Surgeons Trauma Quality Improvement Program. Surg Clin North Am 2012;92:441–54, x–xi.

49. Alali AS, Fowler RA, Mainprize TG, et al. Intracranial pressure monitoring in severe traumatic brain injury: results from the American College of Surgeons Trauma Quality Improvement Program. J Neurotrauma 2013;30:1737–46.

50. Tepas JJ 3rd, Kerwin AJ, Devilla J, et al. Macro vs micro level surgical quality improvement: a regional collaborative demonstrates the case for a national NSQIP initiative. J Am Coll Surg 2014;218:599–604.

51. Carlin AM, Zeni TM, English WJ, et al. The comparative effectiveness of sleeve gastrectomy, gastric bypass, and adjustable gastric banding procedures for the treatment of morbid obesity. Ann Surg 2013;257:791–7.

52. Birkmeyer NJ, Finks JF, Greenberg CK, et al. Safety culture and complications after bariatric surgery. Ann Surg 2013;257:260–5.

The Patient Protection and Affordable Care Act
A Primer for Hand Surgeons

 CrossMark

Joshua M. Adkinson, MD[a], Kevin C. Chung, MD, MS[b],*

KEYWORDS

- Patient Protection and Affordable Care Act ● Affordable Care Act ● Obamacare ● Health care reform
- Hand surgery

KEY POINTS

- The Affordable Care Act has 3 goals: provide health care for all Americans, control costs of health care, and improve the quality of health care.
- To achieve these goals, the government has instituted (1) an individual and business mandate, (2) federal subsidies for health care, (3) new requirements on the health insurance industry, and (4) changes in the practice of medicine.
- The Affordable Care Act also provides new funding for comparative effectiveness research, ties quality measures to reimbursement, and increases taxes on high-income wage earners and medical device manufacturers.

INTRODUCTION

Health care reform in the United States has been a matter of substantial debate in presidential elections since the early 1900s.[1] This evolved from an increasing awareness of patient populations without health insurance. After 8 years of deliberation, the administration of former President Lyndon B. Johnson introduced the Social Security Act in 1965. This bill established the first comprehensive national social insurance program with the creation of the Medicare (for patients over the age of 65) and Medicaid (for individuals or families with low incomes) systems.[2] Despite these landmark efforts, large portions of the population remain without health insurance coverage, and costs of delivering health care are increasing at an unsustainable rate (**Fig. 1**). Proposed solutions to these problems have been either limited or sweeping, but almost always divisive.

On March 23, 2010, President Barack Obama signed into law the Patient Protection and Affordable Care Act (more commonly known as the Affordable Care Act, or ACA).[3] Although the assurance of health care coverage for every American is the prime directive, numerous provisions within the bill aim to control costs and improve health

Supported in part by grants from the National Institute on Aging and National Institute of Arthritis and Musculoskeletal and Skin Diseases (R01 AR062066) and from the National Institute of Arthritis and Musculoskeletal and Skin Diseases (2R01 AR047328-06) and a Midcareer Investigator Award in Patient-Oriented Research (K24 AR053120) (Dr K.C. Chung).
Conflicts of Interest: The authors have no conflicts of interest.
Financial Disclosure: None.

[a] Department of Surgery, Section of Plastic Surgery, University of Michigan Health System, 1500 East Medical Center Drive, Ann Arbor, MI 48109, USA; [b] Section of Plastic Surgery, University of Michigan Medical School, University of Michigan Health System, 2130 Taubman Center, SPC 5340, 1500 East Medical Center Drive, Ann Arbor, MI 48109-5340, USA
* Corresponding author.
E-mail address: kecchung@umich.edu

Hand Clin 30 (2014) 345–352
http://dx.doi.org/10.1016/j.hcl.2014.05.002

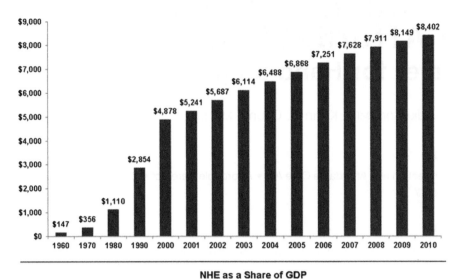

NHE as a Share of GDP

5.2%   7.2%   9.2%   12.5%   13.8%   14.5%   15.4%   15.9%   16.0%   16.1%   16.2%   16.4%   16.8%   17.9%   17.9%

Fig. 1. National health expenditures per capita as a share of gross domestic product, 1960 to 2010. (*Adapted from* Centers for Medicare and Medicaid Services, Office of the Actuary, National Health Statistics Group. Available at: http://www.cms.gov/Research-Statistics-Data-and-Systems/Statistics-Trends-and-Reports/NationalHealthExpendData/ NationalHealthAccountsHistorical.html [see NHE summary including share of GDP, CY 1960–2010; file nhegdp10.zip]. Accessed April 25, 2014.)

care quality in the United States (**Box 1**).[4] The ultimate effects of the ACA on health care in the United States remain an area of considerable uncertainty. Because of the broad scope of this bill, it has far-reaching implications for hand surgeons, including new quality benchmarks and changing reimbursement structures.

The 905-page ACA bill, as originally written, was comprised of 10 titles scheduled to be phased in through Jan. 1, 2018,[5] costing a total of $1.7 trillion (**Box 2**).[6] Title 8 (Community Living Assistance Supports and Services) was abandoned by the

Obama Administration on Oct. 15, 2013, on the grounds that it would not be financially viable.[7] The 5% cosmetic surgery tax in Title 9 was also subsequently repealed, as it was felt to disproportionately affect the middle class and women.[8] There have been many other modifications to the ACA since initial implementation, and this article attempts to provide the most current account of the bill.

KEY ASPECTS OF THE ACA
Access

The ACA is estimated to increase the number of Americans with health insurance by 32 million by 2019.[9] There are multiple avenues through which the ACA attempts to achieve this goal. The most notable measure is by expanding Medicaid eligibility to Americans in a wider income bracket; this alone is estimated to result in 16 to 18 million newly insured Americans.[10] Medicaid eligibility will be expanded to up to 133% of the poverty line. Further, tax credits will be available for the purchase of health insurance for people between with incomes between 100% and 400% of the poverty line.[9] The ACA also limits insurance exclusions, prevents the use of lifetime caps on insurance, makes it illegal to deny insurance coverage for those with preexisting conditions, and allows insurance coverage for children on parental plans up to the age of 26.[9]

Box 1
ACA goals and components

Goals of ACA

- Provide health care for all Americans
- Control costs of health care
- Improve the quality of health care

Essential Components of ACA

- Individual and business mandate
- Federal subsidies for health insurance for uninsured patients
- Extensive new requirements on health insurance industry
- New regulations on the practice of medicine

Box 2
The 10 titles of the ACA

Number	Title	Principal Effects
I	Quality, Affordable Health Care for all Americans	Removal of coverage exclusions based on preexisting conditions, gradual elimination of fee-for-service vs prevention and diminished inpatient and procedure-based care
II	The Role of Public Programs	State-based opt out of Medicaid, Disproportionate Share Hospital program elimination, requirement of essential health benefits
III	Improving the Quality and Efficiency of Health Care	Health care that is more efficient, effective, and patient-centered; implementation of electronic health records and integration of health care databases; medical technology targeted as primary factor for rising costs, especially technology that does not increase health care value; formation of an independent payment advisory board; drive to reorganization of care (accountable care organizations and integrated departments) will affect surgeons
IV	Prevention of Chronic Disease and the Improvement in Public Health	Refocusing health care on prevention of disease, with implications for surgeons
V	Health Care Workforce	Currently, National Health Care Workforce Commission not funded (held up in the US House of Representatives), significant effect on surgical subspecialists if not convened
VI	Transparency and Program Integrity	Addressing health care cost inefficiency and fraud, sunshine provision for physician payment reporting, Patient-Centered Outcomes Research Institute support of research on comparative effectiveness
VII	Improving Access to Innovative Medical Therapies	New Food and Drug Administration regulatory pathways, most profound opportunity is in just-in-time clinical research based on national databases
VIII	Community Living Assistance Supports and Services (CLASS)	This title was abandoned by the Obama administration on Oct. 15, 2013
IX	Revenue Provisions	This title finances approximately half of the ACA, factors affecting hand surgeons are new Medicare taxes on high-income wage earners and new taxes on pharmaceutical and medical technology device manufacturers
X	Strengthening Quality, Affordable Health Care for All Americans	Amendments and additions to Titles I to IX, passed as the Health Care and Education Reconciliation Act signed on March 30, 2010

Adapted from Ferguson TB Jr, Babb JA. The Affordable Care Act: implications for cardiothoracic surgery. Semin Thorac Cardiovasc Surg 2013;25(4):282; with permission.

Beginning in 2014, individuals are required to purchase health insurance (ie, the individual mandate).[11] Failing to obtain insurance coverage will lead to a fine that begins at $95 or 1% of taxable income in 2014. This increases in 2016 to a maximum of $695 for individuals (3 times that for families) or 2.5% of income, whichever is greater.[10] Beginning in 2015, employers with at least ≥100 employees will pay a fine if they do not offer minimum-value, employee-only coverage for any of their workers (ie, the employer mandate).[12] The employer mandate will be delayed until 2016 for businesses with between 50 and 99 employees. To minimize the economic impact on small businesses, these companies may apply for the Small Business Health Care Tax Credit.[13] Penalties resulting from these mandates are anticipated to provide a substantial source of revenue to pay for the ACA.

A state-based health care exchange was implemented in 2014. These exchanges are marketplaces where uninsured individuals and businesses can comparison shop for insurance policies.[3] Variability in health care exchange prices are allowed to vary based only upon patient age, geographic area, family composition, and tobacco use. Further, the insurance industry must use 85% of premiums directly for costs of delivering medical care,[10] and must provide rebates to enrollees if they spend less than 85% on health care as opposed to administrative costs.[14]

Cost

Providing care to current and new Medicare and Medicaid enrollees will come at a considerable cost. Estimates indicate that the Centers for Medicare and Medicaid Services (CMS) will reduce payments to hospitals by $158 billion over 10 years to help defray the cost of the newly insured.[9] Overall health expenditures are projected to decrease by $600 billion over the same time frame.[15] The authors of the law sought to finance nearly half of the cost of the ACA through Title IX provisions. These include new Medicare taxes on high-income wage earners and new taxes on pharmaceutical manufacturers, health insurance providers, and medical device manufacturers. The ACA does not mandate fee restructuring for service reimbursement, but does give the Secretary of Health and Human Services authorization to adjust misvalued fee schedules or procedures and services that have experienced high growth or advances in technology.[9] Changes in payment structures will clearly influence how physicians practice and how care is delivered. Despite the American College of Surgeons' (ACS) recommendation to institute potentially cost-saving medical liability reform with the passage of the ACA, no provisions were included.[16] The implementation of independent panels and regulatory reforms are other ACA strategies to save money.

Independent Payment Advisory Board

The Independent Payment Advisory Board (IPAB) is a board of impartial experts charged with establishing specific target growth rates for Medicare and ensuring that Medicare expenditures stay within these limits. This board is comprised of 15 members appointed by the president for a 6-year term.[17] Members are supposed to be nationally recognized experts in health finance, payment, economics, actuarial science, or health facility and health plan management, and to represent providers, consumers, and payers.[3] There is no mandate for a health care provider (eg, a physician or nurse) to be present on the board, and there is no

congressional authority over the IPAB. However, Congress may increase Medicare funding independently through legislation. This IPAB is prevented from reducing Medicare benefits, raising premiums or taxes, or rationing care. The IPAB is not, however, prohibited from cutting payments for physicians.[17] It is clear that a disproportionate share of these savings will come from surgical services relative to the rest of medicine.[18]

Regulatory reform and combating waste

The US healthcare system is the world's largest and most inefficient information enterprise.[19] In 2009, Thomson-Reuters estimated that the system wastes between $505 and $850 billion annually, reflecting one-third of the nation's healthcare bill.[20] This occurs despite the annual investment of almost $170 billion in health services regulation.[21] The elimination of paper-based medical records in favor of electronic systems alone is estimated to save hospitals and physician practices $371 billion and $142 billion, respectively, over 15 years.[19] Other approaches to combating waste include increased federal sentences (by 20%–50%) for health care fraud over $1 million and enhanced screening (eg, license checks, site visits) of providers who pose a higher risk of fraud.[6] A controversial change in the law now states that a person need not have actual knowledge of this section or specific intent to commit a violation of this section in order to be charged with health care fraud.[5] To avoid unintentional health care fraud and a possible audit, providers should (1) avoid copying and pasting notes (cloning) in electronic medical records, (2) only document services they actually provide and avoid upcoding, (3) and always review billing practices to ensure compliance.

Quality

In 2013, the CMS began to distribute a total of $850 million to hospitals as a reward for meeting a series of quality measures.[9] These funds were generated by reducing the diagnosis-related group (DRG) payments for all hospitals, and then redistributing the savings based on hospital performance. Under the controversial inpatient Value-Based Purchasing Program (VBPP), hospitals are assessed by means of 12 clinical quality measures in 6 domains (patient and family engagement, patient safety, care coordination, population and public health, efficient use of health care resources, and clinical processes/effectiveness) and a composite measure of patient experience.[22] The VBPP is used to decrease payments to hospital providers not meeting certain quality standards established by the CMS.[16]

Physicians will also be increasingly responsible for submitting quality data to the CMS in exchange for payment. The CMS introduced the Physician Quality Reporting System (PQRS) to deliver incentive to providers who enter quality data for review. In 2014, individual providers who satisfactorily submit PQRS quality measures will qualify to earn an incentive payment equal to 0.5% of their total estimated Medicare Part B Physician Fee Schedule (PFS) reimbursements. As of 2015, however, eligible physicians or group practices not submitting PQRS data will be paid 1.5% less (2.0% less in 2016) than the Medicare PFS for that service.[23]

In addition to direct tracking of hospital and individual provider quality measures, quality improvement was addressed in the ACA via the formation of various agencies. The aims of these new entities are to examine current and future strategies for health care delivery and payment, as well as comparative effectiveness of currently available treatments. Further, accountable care organizations (ACOs) were incorporated into the ACA in an effort to give incentives to physicians and hospitals to promote higher-quality, lower-cost healthcare. The ACS, however, warned that caution should be used before using quality and outcomes measures to drive coverage or reimbursement. In 2012, the ACS expressed that quality measures are necessary, but have not been adequately tested and risk-adjusted to serve as a foundation for policy and reimbursement decision-making.[24]

Patient-Centered Outcomes Research Institute

Established in 2010, the Patient-Centered Outcomes Research Institute (PCORI) focuses on funding and promoting comparative effectiveness research.[25] PCORI priorities and criteria are found in (**Box 3**). The anticipated results will assist health care professionals and policy makers in making more informed decisions. As the PCORI has no role in reimbursement decisions, studies funded by this entity are specifically prohibited from examining cost-effectiveness.[26]

Center for Medicare and Medicaid Innovation

In 2010, the ACA established the $10 billion Center for Medicare and Medicaid Innovation with the goal of testing care models that have the potential to improve quality of care and reduce costs.[27] A major focus is on the development of bundled payments for entire episodes of care involving multiple providers across different settings, rather than for discrete services by individual health care providers.[9] As a result, there would be an incentive to coordinate care among providers of different specialties; sharing reimbursement within the

---

Box 3
PCORI priorities and criteria

PCORI Priorities

- Assessment of options for prevention, diagnosis, and treatment
- Improving health care systems
- Communication and dissemination research
- Addressing disparities
- Accelerating PCOR and methodological research

PCORI Criteria

- Impact on the health of individuals and populations
- Improvability via research
- Inclusiveness of different populations
- Addresses current gaps in knowledge/variation in care
- Impact on health care system performance
- Potential to influence decision making
- Patient-centeredness
- Rigorous research methods
- Efficient use of research resources

---

confines of this model is an issue that has yet to be clarified.

Accountable care organizations

ACOs are networks of health care providers that assume accountability for coordination and delivery of effective, high-quality care through a more efficient use of resources.[28] This new patient care model arose in the 1990s in response to the inability of the sustainable growth rate (SGR) to limit spending growth on physician services.[29] The ACA outlines specific requirements that must be met to be designated as an ACO.[30] These criteria can be found in (**Box 4**). Unique features of ACOs include the fact that patients can choose their own providers, keep their insurance, and stay in the Medicare program. By achieving quality improvements and slowing resource utilization, ACOs are remunerated by CMS at an amount equal to a percentage of money saved through cost efficiency.[28] There are currently more than 350 ACOs participating in Medicare.[31] According to CMS estimates, ACO implementation through the ACA is estimated to lead to savings of $470 million from 2012 to 2015.[32] Importantly, 7 of the original 32 pioneer ACOs, including the authors' institution (the University of Michigan), have dropped out of the program, because no savings were realized in 2012.[33]

> **Box 4**
> **Criteria summary for designation as an ACO**
>
> - Express willingness to be accountable for quality, cost, and overall care of Medicare beneficiaries for minimum of 3 years
> - Minimum of 5000 Medicare beneficiaries with a strong core of primary care physicians
> - Legal structure to receive and allocate payments
> - Report on quality, cost, care coordination measures, and meet patient-centeredness criteria

IMPACT OF ACA POLICIES ON HAND SURGEONS

In addition to the innumerable changes already occurring in the health care landscape as a result of the passage of the ACA, many provisions have direct implications for current and future hand surgeons.

Graduate Medical Education

With the signing of the ACA, the government took on a new obligation to ensure millions of people have access to health care. These newly insured patients will seek care from physicians just as funding for graduate medical education (GME) has stagnated. As a result, it is doubtful that there will be a sufficient number of residency positions available to train the necessary future physician workforce.[34,35] This is particularly worrisome for surgical subspecialties, because nearly all efforts at increasing GME funding are directed at primary care.

Payments

Primary care physicians are slated to receive a 10% Medicare bonus for 5 years (2011–2015) under the direction of the ACA. A similar bonus was provided to general surgeons practicing in underserved areas.[34] Conversely, there is a mandated reduction in payments for all other surgical services and the elimination of the disproportionate share hospital (DSH) program payments by Medicare and Medicaid.[9] A DSH is a facility that treats a disproportionate number of indigent patients. The program sought to encourage these hospitals to continue to provide quality services to vulnerable patients by providing funding for uncompensated care.[36] This situation is made more complex by the fact that 24 states have opted out of the Medicaid expansion (these states will lose the benefit of both the DSH and additional Medicaid-covered patients).[37] In aggregate, these changes will disproportionately affect surgeons, particularly those who practice in safety net hospitals (ie, facilities that provide a substantial level of care to low-income, uninsured, or vulnerable populations). Lastly, the ACA will restrain revenues from ancillary services (in-office imaging) and through a modified Stark law prohibiting physicians from referring to a hospital in which they have a financial stake.[13]

Tax Increases

With the implementation of the ACA, several new taxes began starting in 2013. Of these, the 2.3% medical device excise tax will likely impact many hand surgeons; this tax is levied on devices ranging from surgical gloves, instruments, plates and screws for osteosynthesis, joint replacement implants, and advanced imaging technology.[38] Costing manufacturers an estimated $7 billion from 2013 to 2015,[39] some have proposed that this tax may result in considerable harm to research, development, and employment in the medical device industry.[40] In 2012, Stryker (Kalamazoo, Michigan) announced that it would lay off more than 1000 employees as a result of the estimated fiscal impact.[41] Further, it is possible that the increasing costs of medical devices may be passed on to patients.

Other newer taxes directly affect many surgeons' business and personal finances. For example, starting in 2013, the Medicare tax on wages increased by 0.9% to a total of 3.8% of income greater than $200,000 for an individual or $250,000 for a married couple filing jointly. Hand surgeons in this income range are also responsible to pay a new 3.8% Medicare tax on capital gains, dividends, and other passive income. Health flexible spending accounts are now limited to a maximum of $2500 annually, whereas the medical expense deduction threshold was increased from 7.5% to 10% of income.[42]

SUMMARY

The ACA is one of the most comprehensive, expensive, and impactful bills signed in the history of the United States. Health insurance coverage is now extended to millions of individuals not previously covered by a health plan. Using a variety of approaches, the ACA attempts to control costs by regulating health care delivery and reimbursement. The many statutes of the ACA will directly impact all current and future hand surgeon practices and incomes through new taxes on high-income earners and requisite adherence to incompletely defined quality standards. Playing an active role in the development of quality benchmarks and comparative effectiveness research, lobbying for increased GME funding and medical liability reform, and developing more efficient ways of delivering high-quality care will help the specialty transition into the future of US health care. Whether these sweeping changes prove fiscally responsible while improving patient care has yet to be determined.

REFERENCES

1. Henry J. Kaiser Family Foundation. Timeline: history of health reform in the US. 2011 [updated 2011]. Available at: http://healthreform.kff.org/flash/health-reform-new.html. Accessed April 22, 2014.
2. Oliver TR, Lee PR, Lipton HL. A political history of Medicare and prescription drug coverage. Milbank Q 2004;82(2):283–354.
3. Manchikanti L, Caraway DL, Parr AT, et al. Patient Protection and Affordable Care Act of 2010: reforming the health care reform for the new decade. Pain Physician 2011;14(1):E35–67.
4. Albright HW, Moreno M, Feeley TW, et al. The implications of the 2010 Patient Protection and Affordable Care Act and the Health Care and Education Reconciliation Act on cancer care delivery. Cancer 2011; 117(8):1564–74.
5. H.R. 3590. Patient Protection and Affordable Care Act. Washington, DC: US House of Representatives; 2010. Available at: http://frwebgate.access.gpo.gov/cgi-in/getdoc.cgi?dbname=111_cong_bills&docid=f: h3590enr.txt.pdf. Accessed April 22, 2014.
6. Patient Protection and Affordable Care Act. In: Congress US, Public Law 111-148. Washington, DC; 2010.
7. US Department of Health and Human Services. A Report on the Actuarial, Marketing, and Legal Analyses of the CLASS Program. 2011. Available at: http://aspe.hhs.gov/daltcp/Reports/2011/class/index.shtml. Accessed April 28, 2014.
8. Patel A, Shah A, Singh D, et al. Protecting plastic surgery under the affordable care act. Plast Reconstr Surg 2013;131(2):316e–7e.
9. Talwalkar JA. Potential impacts of the Affordable Care Act on the clinical practice of hepatology. Hepatology 2014;59(5):1681–7.
10. Bredesen P. Fresh medicine: how to fix reform and build a sustainable health care system. 1st edition. New York: Atlantic Monthly Press; 2010.
11. Boninger JW, Gans BM, Chan L. Patient Protection and Affordable Care Act: potential effects on physical medicine and rehabilitation. Arch Phys Med Rehabil 2012;93:929–34.
12. Bokert ME, Hahn A, Nelson AD, et al. Final employer mandate and reporting requirement

13. regulations published: it's time to pay or play. Lexology. Available at: http://www.lexology.com/library/detail.aspx?g=a6ea58bc-9a95-43b9-b2a2-8d671a587bf3. Accessed April 24, 2014.
14. Filson CP, Hollingsworth JM, Skolarus TA, et al. Health care reform in 2010: transforming the delivery system to improve quality of care. World J Urol 2011; 29(1):85–90.
15. Manchikanti L, Hirsch JA. Patient Protection and Affordable Care Act of 2010: a primer for neurointerventionalists. J Neurointerv Surg 2012;4(2):141–6.
16. Cutler DM, Davis K, Stremikis K. The impact of health reform on health system spending. Issue Brief (Commonw Fund) 2010;88:1–14.
17. Britt LD, Hoyt DB, Jasak R, et al. Health care reform: impact on American surgery and related implications. Ann Surg 2013;258(4):517–26.
18. Newman D, Davis CM. The Independent Payment Advisory Board. Congressional Research Service Report for Congress. 2010. Available at: http://assets.opencrs.com/rpts/R41511_20101130.pdf. Accessed April 24, 2014.
19. Ferguson TB Jr, Babb JA. The Affordable Care Act: implications for cardiothoracic surgery. Semin Thorac Cardiovasc Surg 2013;25(4):280–6.
20. Hillestad R, Bigelow J, Bower A, et al. Can electronic medical record systems transform health care? Potential health benefits, savings, and costs. Health Aff (Millwood) 2005;24(5):1103–17.
21. Fox M. Healthcare system wastes up to $800 billion a year. Reuters, 2009. Available at: http://www.reuters.com/article/idUSTRE59P0L320091026. Accessed April 24, 2014.
22. Conover CJ. Health care regulation: a $169 billion hidden treatment. Washington, DC: CATO Institute; 2004. Policy Analysis No. 527.
23. Centers for Medicare and Medicaid Services. Medicare program; hospital inpatient value-based purchasing program. Fed Regist 2011;76(9):2454–91.
24. Centers for Medicare & Medicaid Services (CMS), HHS. Medicare program; revisions to payment policies under the physician fee schedule, clinical laboratory fee schedule & other revisions to Part B for CY 2014; final rule. Fed Regist 2013;78(237): 74229–823.
25. Opelka F. Statement of the American College of Surgeons before the Senate Finance Committee on "Medicare physician payments: perspectives from physicians". 2012. Available at: www.facs.org/hcr/. Accessed April 28, 2014.
26. Selby JV, Beal AC, Frank L. The Patient-Centered Outcomes Research Institute (PCORI) national priorities for research and initial research agenda. JAMA 2012;307(15):1583–4.
27. Patient-centered outcomes research. Available at: http://www.pcori.org/patient-centered-outcomes-research/. Accessed April 24, 2014.

27. Provisions of the Affordable Care Act, by year. Available at: http://www.healthcare.gov/law/about/order/byyear.html. Accessed April 24, 2014.

28. Keegan KA, Penson DF. The Patient Protection and Affordable Care Act: the impact on urologic cancer care. Urol Oncol 2013;31(7):980–4.

29. Brown CA. What's wrong with the SGR. Bull Am Coll Surg 2004;89(10):8–11.

30. Goodney PP, Fisher ES, Cambria RP. Roles for specialty societies and vascular surgeons in accountable care organizations. J Vasc Surg 2012;55(3): 875–82.

31. Edwards ST, Abrams MK, Baron RJ, et al. Structuring payment to medical homes after the Affordable Care Act. J Gen Intern Med 2014. [Epub ahead of print].

32. Department of Health and Human Services, Centers for Medicare & Medicaid Services. Medicare shared savings program: accountable care organizations; proposed rules. Fed Reg 2011;76(212):67802–990.

33. Greene J. UM to drop from Pioneer ACO program, will continue to seek Medicare cost savings. 2013. Available at: http://www.crainsdetroit.com/article/20130716/NEWS/130719840/um-to-drop-from-pioneer-aco-program-will-continue-to-seek-medicare#. Accessed April 28, 2014.

34. Iglehart JK. The uncertain future of Medicare and graduate medical education. N Engl J Med 2011; 365(14):1340–5.

35. Petterson SM, Liaw WR, Phillips RL Jr, et al. Projecting US primary care physician workforce needs: 2010-2025. Ann Fam Med 2012;10(6):503–9.

36. Centers for Medicare and Medicaid Services. Disproportionate Share Hospital (DSH). Available at: http://www.cms.gov/Medicare/Medicare-Fee-for-Service-Payment/AcuteInpatientPPS/dsh.html. Accessed April 28, 2014.

37. Sethi MK, Bozic KJ. Where the rubber meets the road: understanding key changes in the Patient Protection and Affordable Care Act since 2010. Clin Orthop Relat Res 2014;472(4):1086–8.

38. Van de Water PN. Excise tax on medical devices should not be repealed: industry lobbyists distort tax's impact. Center on Budget and Policy Priorities. October 2, 2013. Available at: http://www.cbpp.org/files/2-14-12health.pdf. Accessed April 20, 2014.

39. Barthold TA. Revenue estimates. Congress of the United States: Joint Committee on Taxation. June 15, 2012. Available at: http://waysandmeans.house.gov/uploadedfiles/jct_june_2012_partial_re-estimate_of_tax_provisions_in_aca.pdf. Accessed April 20, 2014.

40. Kramer DB, Kesselheim AS. The medical device excise tax — over before it begins? N Engl J Med 2013;368(19):1767–9.

41. Chiaramonte P. Medical giant Stryker cuts 1,170 jobs. Fox News 2012. Available at: www.foxnews.com/politics/2012/11/16/medical-supply-giant-stryker-corp-makes-pre-emptive-strike-against-pending. Accessed April 22, 2014.

42. Bumpass DB, Samora JB, the AAOS Washington Health Policy Fellows. What can we expect from PPACA in 2013? Healthcare reform moving forward. AAOS Now 2013;7(1).

Patient-Centered Care in Medicine and Surgery
Guidelines for Achieving Patient-Centered Subspecialty Care

Reid W. Draeger, MD, Peter J. Stern, MD*

KEYWORDS

- Patient-centered care • Evidence-based medicine • Shared decision making • Hand surgery

KEY POINTS

- Patient-centered care is based on the principle that equality between physician and patient is mutually advantageous, and is a model of patient care commonly favored by patients over a traditional paternalistic model.
- Patient-centered care has 5 main components: the biopsychosocial perspective, the patient as person, sharing power and responsibility, the therapeutic alliance, and the doctor as person.
- Some aspects of patient-centered care are at odds with the disease-centered principles of evidence-based medicine; however, these two models of care are not mutually exclusive.
- By maximizing quality face-to-face time in patient interactions, devoting visit time to nonmedical aspects of the patient's life, empathizing with the patient, being mindful of one's self as a physician during the physician-patient encounter, and by involving patients in decisions about their care, patient-centered care can be achieved by hand surgeons.

INTRODUCTION

In many instances knowing the person who has the disease is as important as knowing the disease that person has.
—James McCormick, 1996.[1]

The physician-patient relationship has evolved from a paternalistic one to a patient-centered one over the past 2 decades. Though regarded as a valuable tenet of primary care, little has been written on patient-centered care in hand surgery or other surgical subspecialties.

Evidence-based medicine, on the other hand, has become an important aspect of the modern hand surgeon's practice. Though often mentioned in the same context as patient-centered care as a model of practice to which one should ascribe, evidence-based medicine may often be at odds with patient-centered care.[2] An appropriate balance of evidence-based and patient-centered care is necessary for optimal patient care in both general practice and surgical subspecialties.

THE PROGRESSION FROM PATERNALISM TO PATIENT-CENTERED CARE

Throughout history, the physician-patient relationship has depended on the medical situation (the physician's and patient's ability to communicate) and the social scene (the sociopolitical and intellectual-scientific climate) at the time.[3] Eras in

Disclosure Statement: The authors have no conflicts of interest to disclose.
Mary S. Stern Hand Surgery Fellowship, Department of Orthopaedic Surgery, University of Cincinnati, 538 Oak Street, Suite 200, Cincinnati, OH 45219, USA
* Corresponding author.
E-mail address: pstern@handsurg.com

Hand Clin 30 (2014) 353–359
http://dx.doi.org/10.1016/j.hcl.2014.04.006
0749-0712/14/$ – see front matter © 2014 Elsevier Inc. All rights reserved.

hand.theclinics.com

which there was a focus on the religious and supernatural, such as ancient Egypt and medieval Europe, resulted in a more activity-passivity, parent-infant type model of physician-patient interaction.[3,4] Times of enlightenment and democratic thought, such as the Greek enlightenment and the Renaissance era, often resulted in a more guidance-cooperation, parent-adolescent type model of care with some participation by the patient.[3,4] Although there have been instances when more egalitarian, mutual-participation models of care were accepted throughout history, a paternalistic model has always been present to some degree.

Patient-centered care, with a stress on mutual participation by the doctor and the patient, was proposed by Szasz and Hollender[4] in the 1950s and further expanded on by Balint[5] in the 1960s. These theories stressed the belief that equality between persons is mutually advantageous and that the physician-patient relationship itself can have great inherent therapeutic value.[3–6]

THE 5 CORE COMPONENTS OF PATIENT-CENTERED CARE

Building on the foundation laid by Balint,[5] leaders in the field have determined that there are 5 components central to patient-centered care[2,6]: the biopsychosocial perspective, the "patient as person," sharing power and responsibility, the therapeutic alliance, and the "doctor as person."[6,7]

The Biopsychosocial Perspective

The biopsychosocial perspective refers to including general biological, psychological, and social factors when considering and treating a patient's condition. This perspective is in contradistinction to the traditional biomedical model of patient care whereby the patient's signs and symptoms are presented to allow for an accurate diagnosis and then treatment. The biopsychosocial perspective requires the physician to have a "willingness to become involved in the full range of difficulties patients bring to doctors, and not just their biomedical problems."[8]

The Patient As Person

Although the biopsychosocial perspective involves understanding the patient's illness in a broad framework, the patient-as-person principle requires understanding the individual patient's experience of illness. The generalizations of the biopsychosocial perspective lay a solid groundwork for patient-centered care, but using the patient-as-person principle the physician understands the meaning of the illness or condition with respect to an individual patient.[6]

Sharing Power and Responsibility

A key aspect to patient-centered care is the sharing of power and responsibility between the physician and patient. An egalitarian physician-patient relationship differs from the traditional paternalistic approach to medical care espoused in the 1950s, and encourages mutual participation by the physician and the patient in medical care and decision making.[3,4] This branch of patient-centered care has been the focus of much study of shared decision making, which has been championed by some as the central pillar of patient-centered care.[9]

The Therapeutic Alliance

Patient-centered care places value on the physician-patient relationship on the premise that a positive relationship between physician and patient can, in its own right, lead to more positive patient outcomes.[6] The therapeutic alliance focuses on the perception of the patient that the doctor is caring, sensitive, and sympathetic. Positive interactions with a physician undoubtedly improve patients' satisfaction with physician encounters, and may help to improve a patient's results through the placebo effect.[6,10]

The Doctor As Person

The doctor-as-person component of patient-centered care stresses the importance of the personal qualities of the physician on patient interactions. It regards the patient-physician interaction as a fluid one in which each party influences the other.[6] The physician's mannerisms, conscious or unconscious (body language, tone of voice), can engender either positive or negative responses and behaviors in the patient. From the physician's perspective, practicing the doctor-as-person aspect of patient-centered care involves self-awareness of emotional responses during the patient interaction.[11]

DISEASE-CENTERED VERSUS PATIENT-CENTERED: THE DIFFERENCE BETWEEN EVIDENCE-BASED MEDICINE AND PATIENT-CENTERED CARE

Although both evidence-based medicine and patient-centered care are stressed as medical practice models to strive toward, the two philosophies are fundamentally different. Evidence-based medicine is disease-oriented as opposed to the patient-oriented approach of patient-centered care.[2] Clinical trials, which are a mainstay of evidence-based medicine, focus on the evaluation and treatment of a certain disease, not a specific patient. The aggregation of data from multiple patients who meet strict inclusion criteria in these studies helps to further eliminate personal patient traits from the patient pool while focusing on a specific malady.

Evidence-based medicine derives conclusions from homogeneous patient populations. Through standardization of study protocols and minimization of confounding factors, results become more reproducible. These factors, in the classic teaching of the scientific method, strengthen an experiment and, consequently, the evidence obtained from it. However, with more patient homogeneity there may be less applicability to clinical practices, where patient populations are more heterogeneous. Patient-centered care argues that different treatments are necessary for different patients based on patient characteristics other than biomedical ones. Patient-centered care focuses on the individualized treatment of each patient based on more "human" characteristics.

Evidence-based medicine does not account for the importance of human relationships in patient care, which is the central pillar of patient-centered care. Whereas patient-centered care acknowledges that the doctor-patient relationship itself is an important determinant of treatment compliance and outcome, evidence-based medicine ignores the effect that this relationship may have on treatment outcomes.

BALANCING PATIENT-CENTERED CARE AND EVIDENCE-BASED MEDICINE

Evidence-based medicine and patient-centered care need not be mutually exclusive. Evidence-based medicine could become more patient-centered if clinical trials were to incorporate patient preferences into their designs.[2] In turn, patient-centered care could become more evidence based through more studies focusing on reproducible measurement of facets of patient-centered care and their relationship to outcomes.[2] Overall, factoring both evidence-based medicine and patient-centered care into practice, the physician should be able to tailor a discussion of relevant evidence surrounding a patient's condition to fit the patient's psychological and social needs.[12]

GUIDELINES FOR PATIENT-CENTERED CARE IN HAND SURGERY
Maximize Quality Time Spent in Face-To-Face Patient Encounters

The time commitment for patient-centered care is a major barrier in surgical subspecialties. In comparison with primary care physicians, most hand surgeons evaluate a larger number of patients in a smaller amount of budgeted appointment time. Maximization of this limited time can help in achieving patient-centered care in a hand surgery practice.

In a 1999 survey of orthopedic physicians and patients conducted by the American Academy of Orthopedic Surgeons, patients reported that having an orthopedist who "listens to patients" and "spends enough time to listen" were both very important qualities to them.[13] Significantly fewer patients, only 13.3%, indicated that they thought their orthopedist "spent enough time to listen," compared with their primary care physician (31.2%) and chiropractor (25.5%).[13] This impression differed dramatically from how orthopedists perceived their practices, with 71.3% of orthopedists characterizing themselves as "spending enough time to listen" during patient interactions.[13]

Evaluating and treating a patient from a biopsychosocial perspective, considering the patient's "biography" as required by the patient-as-person principle, and sharing power and responsibility with the patient all take a great deal of time commitment by the provider, and may not be feasible for some aspects of hand surgery. However, taking steps to maximize quality face-to-face time spent with each patient can help the physician focus on substantive topics of discussion with the patient.

Patient intake forms that include the patient's current medications and allergies, health history, and review of systems can expedite history taking, so that more time can be spent by the physician and patient on the current ailment in the setting of the individual patient's social situation and on the discussion of treatment options. This interaction can strengthen the therapeutic alliance between physician and patient.

Maximizing time spent with patients may have benefits aside from deepening the physician-patient relationship. A study of musculoskeletal patients found that the duration of an office visit directly correlated with patient satisfaction.[14] Other studies have shown that time spent with patients is valuable and increases patient satisfaction, especially when time is spent on shared decision making.[15] In addition, increasing time spent with patients may correlate with a decreasing rate of medical malpractice claims, although this relationship is less clear. Levinson and colleagues[16] found that for a cohort of primary care physicians, those with no malpractice claims spent appreciably more time with patients during office visits than those with a history of malpractice claims. However, when examining a group of surgeons, no such relationship between patients' visit duration and malpractice claims was found, suggesting that other factors may predict malpractice claims among surgeons, such as their technical results.[16]

Devote a Portion of Each Encounter to Nonmedical Aspects of the Patient's Life

In a busy surgical subspecialty practice, one must be mindful that there is much more to a patient than his or her hand surgery condition. Patients often present "clues", or comments about their personal lives or emotions, during office visits that, when recognized by the physician, can allow for the expression of empathy and strengthen the therapeutic alliance between doctor and patient. Unfortunately, more than 60% of these clues are not recognized by surgeons, and represent missed opportunities to connect with patients.[17]

Documenting aspects of the patient's life outside of the doctor's office can help to remind the busy physician of the reason why a patient truly desires to return to good health. Mentioning these nonbiomedical aspects of the patient's life during office visits can help to build a strong patient-physician alliance and increase the trust of the patient in the physician. Increased patient trust, regardless of the means by which it is achieved, has been linked to better health outcomes in internal medicine.[18] It is likely that a similar relationship exists in other medical fields, including hand surgery.

Make an Effort to Empathize with the Patient

Physician empathy is critical in furthering the therapeutic alliance between the physician and patient, which is a cornerstone of patient-centered care. Increasing patient-perceived empathy has been shown to increase patient satisfaction and compliance.[19] Empathy may have as much bearing on patient satisfaction as the patient's perception of physician expertise.[19] In addition, physician empathy may improve the patient's understanding of information or instructions provided by an orthopedist, which could lead to increased patient compliance.[20] Orthopedists[21] and surgeons, in general,[22] have been identified as lacking compassion and empathy when interacting with patients.

Be Mindful of Yourself

The doctor-as-person facet of patient-centered care acknowledges the importance of characteristics of the physician in influencing physician-patient interaction. Appearance, communication style, and attitude, all of which influence the physician-patient relationship, can all be controlled, at least in part, by the physician.

Patients prefer physicians to be professionally dressed in a white coat, and are more likely to share social or psychological issues with these physicians than with those dressed in casual attire.[23] Dressing professionally may be an easy step toward bring a physician closer to practicing effective patient-centered care.

Tone of voice, which can help to express empathy and openness to the patient, is a valuable tool of the physician. In addition, the physician's tone of voice has been linked to malpractice claims by patients, with physicians having more malpractice claims when they use more dominant tones or a tone with a lack of concern.[24]

The attitude of the physician has a strong influence on the patient's perception of the interaction. When the patient and physician share views on patient-centeredness, patients have been found to be more satisfied.[25] Even if the patient does not share the physician's positive attitude toward patient-centeredness or shared decision making, patients of these physicians have been found to be more satisfied than those of physicians who do not embrace patient-centered care.[26]

Involve Patients in Decision Making About Their Care

Patients tend to have a strong preference to share treatment decisions with their physician.[26,27] In addition, shared decision making has been associated with increased patient compliance with treatment, and with optimized psychosocial and physical outcomes.[12,28–31]

Many conditions treated by hand surgeons lend themselves to shared decision making, particularly chronic conditions for which there is no superior treatment.[9] An example is Dupuytren disease, a chronic condition for which urgent treatment is almost never indicated. Lack of a need for urgent treatment allows the physician to foster a strong patient-physician relationship before the patient and physician jointly arrive at a treatment plan.

Shared decision making may be less applicable to acute conditions. Such conditions may often be associated with a clearly superior treatment. For example, compartment syndrome is best treated with fasciotomy to prevent muscle death; an abscess is best treated with irrigation and debridement.

However, acuity of conditions alone does not eliminate the possibility of practicing patient-centered care. Distal radius fractures can be treated both surgically and nonsurgically.

Individualizing treatment to each patient's social circumstances and lifestyle can help maximize excellent results. For example, an intra-articular distal radius fracture in an elderly homemaker might be best treated with open reduction and internal fixation with a volar locking plate if the patient leads an active lifestyle, whereas the injury might be better treated with closed reduction and casting if the patient leads a sedentary life.

Putting shared decision making into practice involves 3 actionable steps: (1) introducing choice, (2) describing options and providing information, and (3) helping patients explore preferences and make decisions.[32] Initially, patients must be informed that reasonable options for treatment exist. Stress should be placed on the importance of respecting individual patient preferences and the role of uncertainty in medicine (ie, therapeutic outcomes may be unpredictable). Second, the treatment options, with pros and cons of each, are presented. Patient education materials can be helpful for conveying this information. Options should be clearly listed in a format understandable by the patient, and can be accompanied by information on potential harms and benefits of each treatment. Finally, the physician elicits patient preferences to help facilitate the patient's treatment decision, and gives the patient an appropriate amount of time to make a decision.

The authors have found that the use of patient education materials can be helpful in guiding shared decision making. Patient education materials for Dupuytren contracture are shown in **Table 1**. These materials clearly list treatment options, and the advantages and disadvantages associated with each. Depending on a patient's health literacy level, during an office visit patients are allowed to review these materials independently or with guidance.

It should be noted that not all patients desire the same level of involvement in decision making about their care. Elderly patients may be more accustomed to paternalism in the doctor-patient relationship, and may be more comfortable with its practice.[12] Bastiaens and colleagues[33] found that although elderly patients generally want to be involved in care decisions, their involvement centers less around making an actual treatment decision more on receiving information from their physician and approving the physician's treatment decision. In addition, those with lower health literacy may be less comfortable making decisions about their treatment.[28] Special consideration must therefore be given to these patient populations. Part of the practice of patient-centered care involves determining a patient's willingness and desire to participate in shared decision making, and tailoring the consultation to this desire.

Table 1
An example of patient education material for Dupuytren contracture, aimed at fostering shared decision making between physician and patient

		Treatment Option		
	Monitor	**Collagenase Enzyme**	**Needle Aponeurotomy**	**Open Fasciotomy (Excision of Cord)**
Location		Office	Operating room/office	Operating room
Method		Day 1: inject Day 2: manipulate One joint at a time Up to 3 injections	Needle used to break up cord	Cord removed surgically
Anesthesia		None to local	Local	Regional or general
Cost		~$3000 per injection (insurance verification)	Surgeon/facility fees	Surgeon/anesthesiologist/ facility fees
Recovery		5–10 d	<7 d	6–12 wk (therapy)
Complications		Skin bruising/tears Allergic reactions Tendon injury Failure (5%)	Skin tears Tendon injury Nerve injury Failure (<2%)	Stiffness Wound-healing problems Nerve injury Vessel injury
Amount of correction		Can be incomplete	Can be incomplete	Can be incomplete
Recurrence (age-dependent)		Probably equal to needle or surgery after 3 y	Variable degree	50% at 10 y (may not require more surgery)

SUMMARY

Overall, patient-centered care can be achieved by hand surgeons, and need not be at odds with evidence-based medicine. Personal reflection by physicians on their interactions, habits, and communication style with patients may yield valuable information and improve patient-centered care. In addition, being in touch with patients' psychological and social needs as well as their biomedical ones can allow for the tailored interpretation and presentation of evidence to patients to facilitate shared decision making. Although more studies on patient-centered care and outcomes are needed, dedication to patient-centered care by hand surgeons likely will result in greater satisfaction of both patients and physicians.

REFERENCES

1. McCormick J. Death of the personal doctor. Lancet 1996;348:667–8.
2. Bensing J. Bridging the gap. The separate worlds of evidence-based medicine and patient-centered medicine. Patient Educ Couns 2000;39(1):17–25.
3. Kaba R, Sooriakumaran P. The evolution of the doctor-patient relationship. Int J Surg 2007;5(1):57–65.
4. Szasz T, Hollender M. A contribution to the philosophy of medicine: the basic model of the doctor-patient relationship. AMA Arch Intern Med 1956;97:585–92.
5. Balint E. The possibilities of patient-centered medicine. J R Coll Gen Pract 1969;17(82):269–76.
6. Mead N, Bower P. Patient-centredness: a conceptual framework and review of the empirical literature. Soc Sci Med 2000;51(7):1087–110.
7. Mead N, Bower P, Hann M. The impact of general practitioners' patient-centredness on patients' postconsultation satisfaction and enablement. Soc Sci Med 2002;55(2):283–99.
8. Stewart M, Brown J, Weston W, et al. Patient-centred medicine: transforming the clinical method. London: Sage; 1995.
9. Barry MJ, Edgman-Levitan S. Shared decision making–pinnacle of patient-centered care. N Engl J Med 2012;366(9):780–1.
10. Crow R, Gage H, Hampson S, et al. The role of expectancies in the placebo effect and their use in the delivery of health care: a systematic review. Health Technol Assess 1999;3(3):1–96.
11. Winefield H, Murrell T, Clifford J, et al. The search for reliable and valid measures of patient-centredness. Psychol Health 1996;11(6):811–24.
12. Taylor K. Paternalism, participation and partnership - the evolution of patient centeredness in the consultation. Patient Educ Couns 2009;74(2):150–5.
13. Frymoyer JW, Frymoyer NP. Physician-patient communication: a lost art? J Am Acad Orthop Surg 2002;10(2):95–105.
14. O'Neill J, Williams JR, Kay LJ. Doctor-patient communication in a musculoskeletal unit: relationship between an observer-rated structured scoring system and patient opinion. Rheumatology (Oxford) 2003;42(12):1518–22.
15. Dugdale DC, Epstein R, Pantilat SZ. Time and the patient-physician relationship. J Gen Intern Med 1999;14(Suppl 1):S34–40.
16. Levinson W, Roter DL, Mullooly JP, et al. Physician-patient communication. The relationship with malpractice claims among primary care physicians and surgeons. JAMA 1997;277(7):553–9.
17. Levinson W, Gorawara-Bhat R, Lamb J. A study of patient clues and physician responses in primary care and surgical settings. JAMA 2000;284(8):1021–7.
18. Lee YY, Lin JL. The effects of trust in physician on self-efficacy, adherence and diabetes outcomes. Soc Sci Med 2009;68(6):1060–8.
19. Kim SS, Kaplowitz S, Johnston MV. The effects of physician empathy on patient satisfaction and compliance. Eval Health Prof 2004;27(3):237–51.
20. Chu CI, Tseng CC. A survey of how patient-perceived empathy affects the relationship between health literacy and the understanding of information by orthopedic patients? BMC Public Health 2013;13:155.
21. Tongue JR, Epps HR, Forese LL. Communication skills. Instr Course Lect 2005;54:3–9.
22. Levinson W, Chaumeton N. Communication between surgeons and patients in routine office visits. Surgery 1999;125(2):127–34.
23. Rehman SU, Nietert PJ, Cope DW, et al. What to wear today? Effect of doctor's attire on the trust and confidence of patients. Am J Med 2005;118(11):1279–86.
24. Ambady N, Laplante D, Nguyen T, et al. Surgeons' tone of voice: a clue to malpractice history. Surgery 2002;132(1):5–9.
25. Krupat E, Rosenkranz SL, Yeager CM, et al. The practice orientations of physicians and patients: the effect of doctor-patient congruence on satisfaction. Patient Educ Couns 2000;39(1):49–59.
26. Carlsen B, Aakvik A. Patient involvement in clinical decision making: the effect of GP attitude on patient satisfaction. Health Expect 2006;9(2):148–57.
27. Little P, Everitt H, Williamson I, et al. Preferences of patients for patient centred approach to consultation in primary care: observational study. BMJ 2001;322(7284):468–72.
28. Youm J, Chenok KE, Belkora J, et al. The emerging case for shared decision making in orthopaedics. Instr Course Lect 2013;62:587–94.
29. Greenfield S, Kaplan SH, Ware JE Jr, et al. Patients' participation in medical care: effects on blood sugar

control and quality of life in diabetes. J Gen Intern Med 1988;3(5):448–57.

30. Griffin SJ, Kinmonth AL, Veltman MW, et al. Effect on health-related outcomes of interventions to alter the interaction between patients and practitioners: a systematic review of trials. Ann Fam Med 2004; 2(6):595–608.

31. Lee YY, Lin JL. Do patient autonomy preferences matter? Linking patient-centered care to patient-physician relationships and health outcomes. Soc Sci Med 2010;71(10):1811–8.

32. Elwyn G, Frosch D, Thomson R, et al. Shared decision making: a model for clinical practice. J Gen Intern Med 2012;27(10):1361–7.

33. Bastiaens H, Van Royen P, Pavlic DR, et al. Older people's preferences for involvement in their own care: a qualitative study in primary health care in 11 European countries. Patient Educ Couns 2007;68(1):33–42.

Clinical Practice Guidelines
What Are They and How Should They Be Disseminated?

Brent Graham, MD, MSc, FRCSC

KEYWORDS

- Practice guidelines • Evidence-based medicine • Practice variation • Guideline dissemination

KEY POINTS

- Clinical practice guidelines use rigorous methods to find, evaluate, and summarize the literature into a series of points that should help guide clinicians in their management of patients.
- Clinicians are often reluctant to implement the recommendations of practice guidelines and the reasons for this vary with the topic and with the practice context.
- Multiple strategies to overcome the barriers preventing implementation should be used together and be selected from the particular characteristics of the target clinician population.

The evidence-based practice movement that started in the 1980s had at its foundation the idea that outcomes would improve if patients were managed using principles developed from medical knowledge accumulated from a body of methodologically sound clinical research. Clinical practice guidelines (CPGs) sought to summarize this medical evidence into general management pathways that clinicians could use to provide patients with the best care possible. However, despite this seemingly laudable objective, CPGs in general have had, in most instances, a modest impact on day-to-day practice. In some cases CPGs have been essentially ignored by most clinicians. The reasons for the failure of CPGs to influence practice are varied but, before examining these, it is important to understand how CPGs are developed (although these methods continue to evolve) and what they represent.

In hand surgery, CPGs have been developed in recent years by the American Academy of Orthopedic Surgeons (AAOS) for the treatment of distal radius fractures,[1] the diagnosis of carpal tunnel syndrome (CTS),[2] and the treatment of CTS.[3] The process for guideline development follows a prescribed series of steps, the goal of which is to produce recommendations that are based on a systematic review of the literature. The CPG Workgroup consists of a panel of medical experts from a variety of clinical backgrounds pertinent to the condition under consideration. This characteristic of the CPG development approach is important and often overlooked. Having the participation of multiple stakeholders minimizes the risk of the recommendations being biased by a specific point of view associated with a particular clinical specialty.

Once the workgroup has been established, the next step is to have the members produce simulated recommendations, that reflect the areas that are thought to be important to developing a useful guideline and help to define the scope of the final document. These simulated recommendations are then used to search the relevant literature. In the case of CPGs produced by AAOS, this

The author has nothing to disclose.
Hand Program, Department of Surgery, University of Toronto, University Health Network, 399 Bathurst Street, East Wing 2-425, Toronto, Ontario M5T 2S8, Canada
E-mail address: brent.graham@uhn.ca

Hand Clin 30 (2014) 361–365
http://dx.doi.org/10.1016/j.hcl.2014.04.007
0749-0712/14/$ – see front matter © 2014 Elsevier Inc. All rights reserved.

literature search is performed by a team of staff members with an epidemiologic background, together with a medical librarian. Workgroup members can also suggest the inclusion of articles that may not be included in the literature search. In general, the focus is on using the literature with the highest level of evidence. If there seems to be a reasonable body of evidence at level II or higher, level III literature is not included unless there is a large volume of potentially important information with this level of evidence. This approach is consistent with the goal of basing the final recommendations on the best possible evidence. The outcomes in the included studies are usually focused on patient-derived measures, consistent with the concept that patient-focused outcomes are the most important.

The next step is to summarize the literature for the workgroup. This is also a task that is usually performed by trained epidemiologists. In the case of the AAOS CPG on CTS treatment, a team of 6 individuals each reviewed 94 articles that were eventually included from an initial pool of more than 300 publications. The data from each article were extracted by each of these 6 individuals and then subjected to statistical analysis appropriate to the measures being evaluated. If possible, comparisons of treatments are summarized, although in many instances the power of the studies precludes this approach. The objective of this phase of CPG development is to analyze the best available data so that a recommendation can be made.

Once the available evidence regarding a recommendation has been reviewed, a consensus of the workgroup members is then sought using nominal group techniques. The use of nominal group methods allows a consensus to be obtained according to preset rules that require secret voting. A single persuasive group member cannot unduly influence the consensus. If there is agreement on the recommendation, it is accepted without further discussion. If there is disagreement among the workgroup members, further discussion is undertaken before a second vote is taken. If a consensus is not reached after a second vote, the recommendation is rejected. The strength of the recommendation, once established, is based on the quality of the evidence and this is expressed together with the recommendation.

WHY DO PHYSICIANS NOT USE CPGS?

Implementation of CPGs by clinicians may be poorer than expected despite the methodologically rigorous process in the CPG development. For example, the Scandinavian Guidelines for the Initial management of Minimal, Mild and Moderate Head Injuries were developed to help physicians caring for these patients and to provide them with safe care that was also cost-effective. The guideline sought to help decision making for patients requiring hospital admission and CT scanning, which are the main drivers of cost. In a sample of more than 500 patients, physicians at their institution complied with the guidelines in only 50% of cases.[4] McGlynn and colleagues[5] reported that overall adherence to evidence-based CPGs published between1998 and 2000 averaged 55%.

The process for developing most CPGs is fully transparent, prospectively planned, and methodologically rigorous. The only recommendations that are adopted are those based solely on the literature and that are supported by a consensus of experts from a broad spectrum of clinical backgrounds. Why then do CPGs sometimes fail to gain traction among clinicians? The reasons are varied and well established. The factors behind the failure of CPGs to influence clinical practice have been studied extensively and have been understood to a greater or lesser extent for almost as long as CPGs have been available. These factors were summarized by Cabana and colleagues[6] in an extensive review of studies of barriers to the implementation of CPGs. These investigators classified the barriers to implementation into 7 broad categories.

Lack of Awareness

Although this varied widely among the studies examined, a lack of awareness was identified to be as high as 84%. In around 80% of the studies, at least 10% of the respondents were unaware of the guidelines.

Lack of Familiarity

These studies tended to indicate that, although there was awareness of the guidelines, familiarity with their content was lacking in a large proportion (a median of 56% of respondents). Overall lack of familiarity was more common than lack of awareness.

Lack of Agreement

The percentage of respondents to the various studies who indicated a lack of agreement with the guidelines was highly variable and seemed to be at least partly linked to the nature of the guideline's recommendation. For example, 91% of respondents to a survey evaluating a guideline published by the American Academy of Pediatrics related to indications for the use of ribavirin indicated that their reason for not using the guideline was disagreement with its recommendations. At the other end of the spectrum, only 1% of respondents indicated disagreement with the recommendations of an American Cancer Society guideline on clinical breast examination.

Lack of Self-efficacy

Self-efficacy relates to individuals' perceptions of their ability to perform a particular activity, which has been reported to be important in determining whether or not a given behavior will be initiated.[7] This barrier was reported to be important to CPG implementation in 68% of the surveys reviewed by Cabana and colleagues.[6]

Lack of Outcome Expectancy

When physicians think that the goal of the guideline is unlikely to be met, they are less likely to implement the recommendations. Cabana and colleagues stated: "...since physicians see patients individually, they may not discern success at the population level. Overlooking population-level successes can negatively influence outcome expectancy and lead to non-adherence." In almost 90% of the surveys reviewed, this was an important factor in nonadherence for at least 10% of respondents.

Inertia of Previous Practice

All of the studies found that at least 10% of respondents listed this as a barrier to implementation of guideline recommendations.

External Barriers

External barriers may include simple factors such as the time required to put into practice a particular recommendation. Guidelines may be perceived as difficult to implement or physicians may think that recommendations conflict with patient preferences. In addition, implementation of guidelines may also be affected by practice circumstances, such as facilities that are under the control of an institution, increased costs, decreased reimbursement, or the perception of an increased vulnerability to liability.

Similar findings have been reported by Farquhar and colleagues,[8] who reviewed more than 11,600 responses to questions on 7 themes related to implementation of CPGs. These themes ranged from their role as sources of advice, educational tools, and mechanisms to improve quality of care and reduce health care costs to their impact as causes of increased liability risk and loss of physician autonomy. More than 70% of respondents indicated that guidelines were helpful as sources of advice, good educational tools, and intended to improved quality of care; 53% of respondents saw guidelines as intended to reduce health care–related costs. Substantial percentages of respondents considered CPGs to be negative, 41% thought CPGs increased medicolegal vulnerability, 34% thought they diminished physician autonomy, and 30% thought they were too inflexible to apply to individual patients.

The concern that CPGs increase risk of medicolegal action bears closer examination. There is little evidence that CPGs have been used in this way. Farquhar and colleagues[8] quoted a study by Brushwood[9] indicating that CPGs were used to prove negligence in less than 7% of medicolegal cases in the United States. The standard of care is usually defined by what would be performed under usual circumstances by most physicians. If this standard conforms to a CPG, a physician should feel protected rather than threatened by adherence to the recommendations. If a practice is outside an evidence-based guideline with which most clinicians agree, then it may represent suboptimal care.

In 2014, physicians obtain information in ways that are different from even 10 years ago; however, some of these factors are still likely to be important barriers to guideline implementation many years after these early reports. An especially important cause of a failure to adhere to CPGs is disagreement with the recommendations. Now that physicians have a greater awareness of evidence-based practice than they might have had 20 years ago, a common concern is the poor level of evidence on which CPG recommendations are based. The AAOS recommendations are accompanied by a grade that reflects the level of evidence leading to the recommendation. A poor level of evidence leads to a weak grade for the recommendation. In some cases this has led to a failure of clinicians to adopt the recommendations, even though these should be seen as reflecting, at the least, the best available evidence.

HOW AND WHY DO PHYSICIANS CHANGE THEIR PRACTICES?

The ways that physicians change their behavior has been reviewed by Molding and colleagues.[10] They identify 8 key principles that have an important impact on changing physician behavior and they conclude that these factors have to be taken into consideration in the dissemination of evidence-based CPGs:

- Recognition that change in behavior is a process

- Thought leaders (change agents) must identify with the concerns of clinicians who are the targets of CPGs
- Assessment of the readiness to change and the specific barriers to these changes
- The recognition that multiple strategies for change are more effective than any single strategy; education of clinicians must address the domains of knowledge, attitudes, and skill development; education strategies must encourage interaction and participation by clinicians
- Social influences may play an important role
- Environmental support (ie, support by institutions) is important to both initiating change and maintaining the new status quo

The investigators concluded that consideration of these factors should allow the development of effective dissemination strategies that address the specific barriers to change of the target clinician population.

An effective approach to the implementation of guidelines for venous thromboembolism prophylaxis, incorporating many of these ideas, has been reported by Pannucci and colleagues.[11] The key strategy was to first identify champions: individuals particularly committed to the success of the initiative. Two physicians and 1 physician's assistant undertook this role and took responsibility for educating the most important stakeholders, starting with the academic leaders in the institution and continuing with the staff surgeons. Surgical trainees, the main order writers at the institution, and physician's assistants should receive educational sessions separate from the staff physicians. Education continued in the form of monthly e-mail messages and journal clubs on the topic of venous thromboembolism prophylaxis. A risk stratification instrument was used to evaluate patients in preoperative assessment clinics and completion of this was required before any order entry for these patients. Online order entry had also been adopted by the institution, thus facilitating this particular strategy. Compliance with the protocol increased from 10% to 55% during the education phase, before formal adoption of the protocol. Compliance eventually increased to 90% and was maintained at this level 12 months after adoption, even after monthly e-mail reminders had been discontinued 9 months after the study began. Previous studies of implementation of venous thromboembolism prophylaxis protocols indicated that generally compliance ranged from 16% to 64%. Only 1 previous study reported compliance of more than 80%.[12]

SUMMARY

CPGs are intended to improve the care delivered to patients by reducing variation in management and by emphasizing practices that are based on the best available evidence in the literature. They result from a transparent and methodologically rigorous systematic review and analysis of the literature and as a result can be accepted as being free of important bias. If the literature on a given topic is weak or conflicting, the strength of CPG recommendations is limited. However, they still represent a fair and informative distillation of what is known on a given topic. The reasons underlying the failure of physicians to adopt the recommendations contained in CPGs are varied and dictate a similarly varied and multidimensional approach to informing, reminding, and reinforcing clinician behavior.

REFERENCES

1. Lichtman DM, Bindra RR, Boyer MI, et al. Treatment of distal radius fractures. J Am Acad Orthop Surg 2010;18(3):180–9.
2. Keith MW, Masear V, Chung K, et al. Diagnosis of carpal tunnel syndrome. J Am Acad Orthop Surg 2009;17(6):389–96.
3. Keith MW, Masear V, Amadio PC, et al. Treatment of carpal tunnel syndrome. J Am Acad Orthop Surg 2009;17(6):397–405.
4. Heskestad B, Baardsen R, Helseth E, et al. Guideline compliance in management of minimal, mild, and moderate head injury: high frequency of noncompliance among individual physicians despite strong guideline support from clinical leaders. J Trauma 2008;65(6):1309–13.
5. McGlynn EA, Asch SM, Adams J, et al. The quality of health care delivered to adults in the United States. N Engl J Med 2003;348:2635–45.
6. Cabana MD, Rand CS, Powe NR, et al. Why don't physicians follow clinical practice guidelines? A framework for improvement. JAMA 1999;282(15):1458–65.
7. Bandura A. Social foundations of thought and action; a social cognitive theory. Englewood Cliff (NJ): Prentice-Hall; 1986.
8. Farquhar CM, Kofa EW, Slutsky JR. Clinicians' attitudes to clinical practice guidelines: a systematic review. Med J Aust 2002;177:502–6.
9. Brushwood DB. Clinical practice guidelines and the standard of care. Am J Health Syst Pharm 2000;57:159–61.
10. Moulding NT, Silagy CA, Weller DP. A framework for effective management of change in clinical practice: dissemination and implementation of clinical practice guidelines. Qual Health Care 1999;8:177–83.

11. Pannucci CJ, Jaber RM, Zumsteg JM, et al. Changing practice: implementation of a venous thromboembolism prophylaxis protocol at an academic center. Plast Reconstr Surg 2011;128:1085–92.

12. Worel JN. Venous thromboembolism: what is preventing achievement of performance measures and consensus guidelines? J Cardiovasc Nurs 2009;24:S14–9.

Funding Research in the Twenty-First Century
Current Opinions and Future Directions

Lee Squitieri, MD, MS[a], Kevin C. Chung, MD, MS[b],*

KEYWORDS

- Physician-scientists • Mentor • Grant writing • Funding

KEY POINTS

- Physician-scientists have the unique potential to combine scientific insight with clinical perspective to advance the field of medicine, either through basic science, outcomes, or health services research. Their cultivation and preservation are critical to maintaining the United States' position as a world leader in biomedical innovation and shaping the future of medicine in an era of rapid change.
- Although previously immune to the pressures that influence other consumer-related service industries, academic medicine in the twenty-first century will be forced to confront declining reimbursements, universal healthcare, direct-to-patient advertising, patient-rated outcomes, exponential growth in technology, structural changes in organization, and regulatory transformations.
- Mastering all of the traditional elements of clinical practice, teaching, research, and administration may not be possible for future physician-scientists, and establishing clinical and research areas of expertise will be critical to achieve academic excellence and leadership in one's surgical field.
- For young surgeons today to be successful in developing an academic career, they must understand the aforementioned challenges and prepare themselves for a long and committed road to achieving research independence.
- Being able to adapt and learn skills from mentors outside of one's specialty may be a critical element for success in certain environments and may also lead to developing innovative collaborative projects worthy of high-profile grants.
- Residents and junior surgical faculty must also find a way to balance their clinical education with learning the necessary research, administrative, and leadership skills to be competitive.
- Finally, researchers at all levels must realize at the beginning of their career that triumph over this long path requires an incredible amount of sacrifice and hard work along the way. In the current grim environment for grant success, they should not let negative outcomes lead to a loss of morale or momentum, because with the proper planning and guidance they will persevere.

> It was the best of times, it was the worst of times.
>
> —Dickens.[1]

In their recent 2013 National Institutes of Health (NIH) directors' blog, Drs Sally Rockey and Francis Collins quoted the above line from Charles Dickens' *A Tale of Two Cities* in the context of US biomedical research and grant funding.[2] The "best of times" refers to the exponential rapid growth in scientific advancements and research opportunities over the past several years. The "worst of times" reflects the decreasing ability of

---

[a] Division of Plastic and Reconstructive Surgery, Department of Surgery, University of Southern California, 1510 San Pablo Street, Suite 415, Los Angeles, CA 90033, USA; [b] Section of Plastic Surgery, Department of Surgery, University of Michigan Health System, University of Michigan, 2130 Taubman Center, 1500 East Medical Center Drive, Ann Arbor, MI 48109–0340, USA
* Corresponding author.
E-mail address: kecchung@umich.edu

Hand Clin 30 (2014) 367–376
http://dx.doi.org/10.1016/j.hcl.2014.04.002
0749-0712/14/$ – see front matter © 2014 Elsevier Inc. All rights reserved.

the NIH to support all of the vital research that currently makes the United States a world leader in biomedical innovation. The directors project that over the next decade, inflation combined with budget cuts and sequestration could result in a $19 billion loss in research funding.[2] In fact, this year the NIH will be funding 650 fewer research grants than it did last year, resulting in a less than one in six chance of grant applications being funded.[2]

It is well understood that for all academic biomedical researchers, the process of submitting grants and securing research funding is a critical part of advancing one's career.[3–5] Grant awards from the NIH or other specialty organizations elevate a department's standing within their own specialty and within their home institution. Acquisition of extramural funding not only strengthens the department's recruiting ability, but also liberates internal resources for use toward expanding the department or institution. The connection between grant awards and departmental growth is largely responsible for the traditional relationship between publications and grant acquisition with academic promotion and career advancement.[6,7]

However, in the current era of decreasing new grant awards and renewals leading to significantly worse success rates, it is hard for young aspiring physician-scientists to remain optimistic regarding their future in academic medicine.[2] Despite the increasing number of US medical students, the number of graduates desiring to pursue a career in research continues to critically decline.[8,9] Careers in academic medicine are discouraged in the current environment by financial disincentives, ambiguous and inflexible promotional tracks, limited leadership, and a lack of formal exposure or training in medical school.[10–12]

Furthermore, studies have shown that surgeons are less successful than their nonsurgical colleagues in obtaining extramural NIH grants, the most prestigious source of research funding.[13] These sobering realities raise awareness regarding the difficult future for young surgeons endeavoring to succeed in academic medicine, and highlight the importance for today's young surgeon-scientists to prepare and adapt to the inevitably changing climate of research funding. This article provides a primer on developing a successful career as a funded surgeon-scientist and pathways for building a robust research platform worthy of extramural NIH funding in the twenty-first century.

CHOOSING A MENTOR

It is widely accepted among leaders in academic medicine that the first and most important decision a young investigator should make is the selection of a research mentor.[6,7,11,14–22] In general, mentors should have expertise in and commitment to a research area that interests the mentee, and a strong history of publications, grant funding, and successful mentoring.[14] The ideal mentor provides efficient resources, purposeful opportunities, unbiased advice, and protection from distracting forces.[20] Choosing an experienced mentor early in one's academic career is critical in mapping a successful research platform and more important than any individual research project in which the young trainee participates.[14] This is because junior research projects guided by an experienced mentor should serve as a training ground to develop research skills and begin a study portfolio, rather than answer an isolated research question. Early career investigators should select someone within their own institution who understands the unique culture, politics, and promotional tenure policies of the department and institution so that they may help the mentee craft their research portfolio accordingly.[6,7,17] Young researchers should avoid choosing a junior faculty member who does not have the time or experience to mentor an even more junior colleague.[14,18–21] Similarly, they should also avoid senior investigators who are too busy to dedicate the time and effort required to guide an inexperienced junior researcher.[14,18–21] The goal of the mentor-mentee relationship at this stage is for the mentor to provide directed education, training, and career development through small focused projects so that the mentee may collect pilot data and progress toward leadership of larger research proposals worthy of grant funding.

As researchers advance in their career, networking and interdepartmental collaboration become critical components of academic success. Research mentors at this junction should be leaders in the field with access to experienced senior collaborators and knowledge regarding educational and professional opportunities for the mentee.[6,7,14,20] Trainees should learn from their mentors how to assemble, interact, and lead a team of research professionals with various skills and experiences. Mentors should assist the mentee in using the assets of a research team to leverage support for their ideas and obtain grant funding to build a focused research portfolio. Through this process, the mentee learns from the mentor how to define an area of expertise and become established as a leader in the field. The goal of mentorship at the senior level is to teach the trainee how to successfully obtain extramural funding and function independently as the leader of a research team.

Over the course of a research career, a physician-scientist may acquire multiple mentors to fulfill different needs as they professionally mature.[14,17] In fact, some investigators believe that traditional one-on-one mentorship does not provide the breadth of guidance needed to remain competitive in the forthcoming complex environment of research, medical practice, and teaching.[23–25] However, at any stage in one's career, the most important factor when choosing a mentor is the unique professional dynamic and open communication between the mentor and mentee. Mentees should be continuously proactive in their own career development and take responsibility for recognizing, guiding, and facilitating the efforts of the busy mentor.[18] They should identify a person they are compatible with who understands their work habits and skill set and is willing to commit the necessary time to help the mentee build on their strengths and identify what truly interests them. Both parties should critically evaluate the values and work style of the alternate party to understand if working together will be an enjoyable and collaborative experience.[20,21] The productivity, success, and happiness of both parties is contingent on the ability to openly communicate and work cooperatively.

MAPPING A CAREER DEVELOPMENT PATHWAY

At the outset of their career, trainees should recognize that becoming a successful physician-scientist requires an incredible amount of hard work and sacrifice that may at times prolong or delay the development of their clinical practice and personal life.[20] However, in exchange for this dedicated effort, physician-scientists have the remarkable potential to advance the field of medicine and improve the care of millions of patients, all while answering research questions that they truly find interesting. Enthusiastic young investigators should not be intimidated or discouraged by the long road ahead. Rather, they should embrace their passion and meticulously craft their career to best position themselves for academic success.

Once a research mentor is selected, trainees should clearly identify their career goals with their mentor and actively begin to craft a focused research portfolio.[14] It is critical for early investigators to remain concentrated on a specific research theme and sequentially build on prior experiences. Successful mentors help early trainees avoid the trap of working on too many disconnected and haphazard projects with inexperienced collaborators, because they understand that achieving senior-level extramural funding is a long step-wise process that requires focused demonstration of progressive research success over many years. Experienced senior investigators guide their junior colleagues in building a group of interrelated projects with preliminary data worthy of competing for extramural long-term funding, and perhaps ultimately leading to an NIH R01 grant. Successful recipients of these prestigious awards must have a track record of securing and building on the results of prior small grant proposals to produce high-impact results.

In addition to assistance with specific research projects, mentors should also help the mentee obtain formal research training that fits within (or around) their clinical practice or residency/fellowship program.[14,20] For young surgery residents or junior attendings, this critical element of education poses a unique administrative challenge. Unlike other medical specialties with predictable clinical commitments, the rigorous inflexible demands of a surgical career usually require that the mentee find some amount of guaranteed protected time away from clinical activities to adequately develop an area of research expertise.[20,21] This commitment can be extremely difficult to organize because it requires securing a mentored research experience, coverage of clinical responsibilities, and an alternative method of financial income. However, a lack of protected research time has been shown to hamper physician-scientist productivity and ultimate academic success.[20,26] For every 10 hours of clinical work per week, physician-scientists experience a 23% decrease in the odds of obtaining federal or nonprofit grant support.[20,26] Young investigators should be aware that the application process for many funded research mechanisms usually takes 1 to 2 years, and they should discuss their desire to pursue these avenues as early as possible with their program director or faculty advisor.

After securing protected research time, mentorship, and monetary support trainees should perform a gap analysis to identify existing knowledge gaps in a particular area and opportunities for new studies and leadership.[14] Using this foundation, the mentor and mentee should craft a unique clinician-scientist pyramid for success for the mentee (**Fig. 1**).[14] Each layer of the pyramid introduces an additional level of research skill and progressive administrative/leadership responsibilities. Although each mentee will not be able to plan their entire research path in detail at the beginning of their career, they should construct a general plan and review periodic priority lists with their mentor to guide their progress and keep the mentee focused on his or her dedicated research track.[14,20,21]

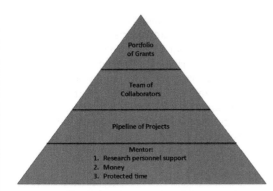

Fig. 1. Physician-scientist pyramid for success. (*From* Lai WW, Vetter VL, Richmond M, et al. Clinical research careers: reports from an NHLBI pediatric heart network clinical research skills development conference. Am Heart J 2011;161:54; with permission.)

Fig. 2 outlines a more in-depth career path for young surgeons including potential timelines for progressive research publications, grant funding, and academic career advancement. Beginning with more simplistic short-term studies, such as case reports, systematic reviews, and literature reviews, the early investigator may work closely with the senior mentor to develop their writing abilities and familiarize themselves with the process of manuscript submission and review. Once these skills are solidified and a chosen area of clinical and research interest has been identified, the junior investigator should progress in the analytical skills necessary for short-term retrospective chart reviews or simple database analyses.[6,14] These research projects may be easily performed over the course of 1 to 2 years for the purpose of

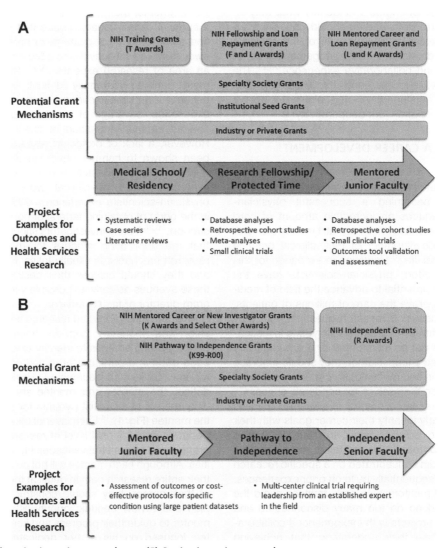

Fig. 2. (*A*) Junior investigator pathway. (*B*) Senior investigator pathway.

collecting pilot data. They are also usually low-budget, less labor intensive, and do not rely on complex collaboration, making them more amenable to medical students, residents, and junior faculty who may need to balance clinical responsibilities without much protected research time or funding support.

As investigators become more advanced, they should aggressively seek protected research time to develop a focused area of research expertise and career path. They should seek formal training in higher level statistics and analytical techniques required to perform complex database analyses, small institutional clinical trials, and meta-analyses. They should also gain experience in effectively communicating with collaborators to develop and troubleshoot ideas, and potentially direct a junior research assistant or statistician. Finally, using their acquired skills and pilot data from initial small studies, the mid-level investigator may attempt to write and submit an entry level grant. This includes developing administrative responsibilities, such as drafting a research budget and timeline, and maturing their analytical foresight to determine sequential research aims and deliverable items.

Traditionally, new investigators have relied on receiving federally funded mentored career development grants, such as K awards or pathway to independence awards, to provide salary support for protected research time.[6,13,15,16,27–29] These grants represent the best mechanism to develop a robust and focused research portfolio over 3 to 5 years, the usual amount of time required for junior faculty to become productive in research and effective as teachers.[22] However, as with all federally funded grants, career development awards are becoming increasingly more competitive. Therefore, given the decreasing rate of grant awards and the time required for each round of grant submission, junior researchers should simultaneously seek alternative career development or seed funding from internal grant mechanisms at their home institution, national specialty agencies, industry sponsors, or private organizations (**Table 1**).[4,14,16]

Early mentored research grants should justify professional career growth for the junior investigator and help him or her become established as an expert in the studied research area and as a future leader in the field.[6,16,27,29] Through these proposals, young trainees should gain experience in various research methodologies, statistical modeling, grant and manuscript writing, team leadership, and administrative budgeting. Examples of potential studies at this stage include single-center prospective clinical trials, large dataset manipulations with complex modeling, and economic analyses. Results of these studies should generate a focused research portfolio with a diverse demonstration of skills that may be used to justify larger, extramural, and independent grant mechanisms.

Once the investigator has successfully used smaller mentored grants to demonstrate leadership and productivity through numerous related first author publications, they may consider applying for an independent grant.[6,16] Independent grants are generally targeted toward established senior investigators and more focused on the actual proposal itself, rather than career development of the study investigator.[16] Logistical planning of these grants is critical and often requires skillful interdisciplinary or multi-institutional collaboration. Furthermore, the results of these studies usually have great impact on the overall medical community. Examples of grants at this stage include multicenter clinical trials, multidisciplinary assessment of complex medical conditions, development and validation of an outcome assessment tool, and linked database analyses to explore national variations in care. During this time, the trainee should also transition to the level of senior investigator and participate on editorial boards of journals and national study sections.[7] Through their funded projects they should also take the opportunity to mentor and teach junior colleagues.[7]

WRITING AND SUBMITTING A GRANT

There are numerous detailed references for young surgeons regarding the finesse of "grantsmanship" and the art of successful grant writing.[15,16,27,28] A detailed review is beyond the scope of this article; however, we provide a brief overview of the key elements of grant success. It is critical for junior investigators to identify potential sources of funding as early as possible, even before the collection of pilot data, so that they may design their preliminary studies accordingly. Investigators should obtain copies of previously funded grants from either experienced mentors or directly from the granting agency to understand the expectations, values, and motivations of each funding source.[16,29,30] This allows researchers to appropriately structure their research aims, methods, and deliverables to fit the desired grant model and timeline. Ideally, a research team and funding source should be identified no later than 12 months before the grant deadline.[29,30] This is to ensure sufficient time for thorough concept development, meticulous detailed study aims and methods, administrative lag time, and sufficient troubleshooting of potential limitations.

Table 1
Types of grant funding

Type of Grant Funding	Description	Examples
Institutional	Smaller less competitive grants generally available through academic institutions Good place to start for young investigators Aim to provide funding to support preliminary work that will lead to larger extramural funding	Specific to academic institution
Private	Rigid guidelines and aims, specific to the mission of the foundation and advancing the care of specific patient populations	Breast Cancer Research Foundation
Industry	Rigid guidelines and aims, specific to advancing the interests of the company	Medical device companies
National specialty societies	Usually provide a range of small funds for junior investigators and large funds for senior investigators Aim to provide funding to support preliminary work that will lead to larger federal funding	American Foundation for Surgery of the Hand
Federal	Most inclusive regarding types of proposals they will fund because 27 different institutes (http://www.nih.gov/icd/) Provide various levels of grant funding for junior and senior investigators	National Institutes of Health Department of Defense US Department of Veterans Affairs

Data from Lai WW, Vetter VL, Richmond M, et al. Clinical research careers: reports from an NHLBI Pediatric Heart Network Clinical Research Skills Development Conference. Am Heart J 2011;161:13–67; and The Plastic Surgery Foundation Researcher Education Committee. Grant writing module. Available at: http://www.thepsf.org/Documents/PSF%20Grant%20Writing%20Module%208.22.13%20FINAL.pdf. Accessed December 15, 2013.

Because of the significant amount of time associated with grant preparation, including conduction of preliminary studies, identification of available resources, building a reliable research team, and writing a proposal, it is wise for early investigators to construct a project that may be widely applied to meet the needs of various grant agencies. This positions the investigator to simultaneously pursue multiple potential funding sources and also forces them to critically evaluate ways in which the chosen research theme may be expanded or revised to accommodate new populations or areas of research interest. For example, the same research idea of evaluating the outcomes of distal radius fractures after an operative intervention may be studied in various patient populations with different research outcomes and implications. However, this research theme needs to be reformatted with a slightly different spin (significance, aims, study population, methods) and

budget when presented before different grant agencies. Each funding source is interested in promoting research that improves the health care of a target patient population, and therefore the same grant needs to be adjusted accordingly to align with the motivations, timeline, and scope of the specific grant.

When writing a grant, researchers should write persuasively and actively with the reviewers in mind.[30] The goal should be to "sell" the research proposal to the reviewers while following the aims of the funding agency and the specific format of the grant.[8,19] Writing and figures should be simple, clear, and understandable to professionals outside of the researcher's chosen specialty.[16,30] This point is critical for small surgical fields that are underrepresented on most grant review committees other than specialty-specific seed grants. Successful grants often have a robust demonstration of pilot data and evidence of a guaranteed data source (eg, animal or patient population, database, or contracted collaboration). The study aims and deliverables must be practical and result in conclusions that will impact the current practice of medicine and design of further research. For mentored career development grants, the proposal must also demonstrate a level of professional growth for the junior mentee.

After an initial draft of the grant is compiled, investigators should seek the review of senior researchers with and without expertise in grant proposals. This round of review is critical because it identifies pitfalls in research methodology and communication. Review from expert colleagues may also highlight potential ways in which the aims and significance of the research study could be expanded in the current grant or future subsequent grants, using results from this study as preliminary data. For many researchers, the process of assembling grant documents for submission and incorporating feedback from senior mentors and reviewers is the most arduous task, because this requires long hours of hard work, administrative savvy, meticulous attention to detail, and a strong commitment to the proposal.

Once these steps are complete, the grant may be submitted. However, the "path to independence" does not end with grant submission or even grant acceptance. If the grant is rejected, researchers should carefully review feedback from the grant agency and modify the proposal for resubmission or submission to an alternative source. Investigators should note that many grant agencies have a limited number of resubmissions per grant proposal. If the grant is accepted by the proposed agency, investigators should not slow down in the face of success. Rather, they should already be working toward their next project or plans for expanding the current results for a related higher-impact proposal, because they already know from prior experience all of the lengthy troubleshooting required to develop high-impact ideas.

CAREER MANAGEMENT AND BALANCING DEMANDS

When developing a research portfolio, many junior academic surgeons are usually at a time in their life when they are also forced to balance life changes, financial debt, and growing clinical responsibility. Managing all of these commitments can be extremely taxing and stressful, leaving little room for the development of essential administrative and leadership skills.[20,22] Many surgery programs have noted a lack in education regarding professional development outside of the clinical arena.[31,32] This has resulted in a generation of young faculty ill prepared to navigate the stressful art of balancing their research careers with a developing clinical practice, teaching responsibilities, and increasing personal commitments.[31,32]

Especially in the current era of massive healthcare reform, young physicians more than ever will depend on administrative and leadership skills to adapt to inevitable changes regarding the organization of healthcare systems and the delivery of patient care. Similarly, physician-scientists will rely on these same skills to build their research laboratory and remain competitive for emerging grant mechanisms. Dedicated time off and formal training for nonclinical professional development are scarce and may not be financially or clinically viable for young surgery residents or attendings. Thus, if unable to attain protected time off for research or administrative duties, junior faculty should learn from their mentors and proactively seek out opportunities to gain experience leading teams, teaching junior colleagues, and communicating or collaborating with professionals outside their chosen specialty.

Young surgeons should also realize that it is near impossible to develop all aspects of one's professional career and personal life simultaneously. The road to a successful and balanced senior academic career is taking advantage of select focused opportunities in a calculated stepwise fashion. Trying to advance in all areas and accomplish a disorganized set of goals at the same time inevitably results in an unsatisfying experience, limited success, and a high risk of physician burn-out. More than one-third of American physicians and 40% of surgeons suffer from professional burn-out, a syndrome categorized by emotional exhaustion, depersonalization, and a low sense of personal accomplishment.[33–36] Burnout among surgeons has been associated with personal dysfunction and physical illness, decreased professional performance, lapses in patient care, and an elevated self-perceived likelihood of leaving academic medicine.[33–35,37] In the face of increasing economic pressure, surgeon-scientists suffer from heightened demands to be productive in all academic arenas. Thus, it is critical for young aspiring physician-scientists to be honest with themselves and with their mentors regarding both their professional and personal aspirations, so that they may pace themselves appropriately and structure their career path accordingly.[20,34]

The concept of work-family balance may be particularly difficult for female surgeons, as they confront the issue of starting a family. Women in surgery experience higher rates of burnout than their male counterparts and increased guilt associated with balancing a career.[20,37] Subsequent to the increased physical demands and emotional pressure associated with raising a family, many female physician-scientists tend to be most productive later in life (50–60 years old).[20] This timeline does not usually fit within the typical academic career trajectory and promotional tenure policy, making it even more difficult for aspiring female academic surgeons to remain committed to their research career. However, dedicated time off for research with a more flexible schedule may afford opportunities for young female surgeons to devote time to personal commitments. Thus, rather than neglect their nonclinical and personal life to advance their research career, female surgery residents and junior attendings should work with their mentor to plan alterative paths to accomplish these goals via protected time away from clinical duties or selection of a clinical or research area that allows flexibility to accomplish their individual goals.[20,34,37]

THE CHANGING CLIMATE OF GRANT FUNDING AND PROMOTIONAL TENURE

There is no doubt that with the increasing competition among mentored career development grants and decreased availability of funds, the traditional pathway toward academic promotion will be redefined in the coming years. To nurture and maintain the academic passion of an increasingly diverse generation of physician-scientists, junior faculty development and tenure policies need to develop alternative career pathways aligned with a variety of scholarship interests.[38] New attendings aspiring to succeed on the physician-scientist track should be encouraged to identify themselves as either basic science researchers, clinical outcomes researchers, or health services researchers. Merit assessment, funding expectations, and distribution of efforts should differ for these categories of researchers and tenure policies may need to accommodate alternative sources of funding and data acquisition. Similarly, to increase retention of female faculty and male faculty with children, who may not peak in their research output until later in life, some have suggested a tenure rollback "Stop-the-Clock" option.[38,39]

The increasing emphasis on patient-driven treatment selection and outcomes has subsequently resulted in the transformation of medicine into a more consumer-driven service industry of the twenty-first century.[23] As the number and value of federally and specialty funded grants continue to decline, the relative influence of private-interest group, industry, and payor-driven grant mechanisms will likely increase. These changes can already be seen with various industry-specialty partnered grants, such as the Plastic Surgery Foundation–Musculoskeletal Transplant Foundation grant offered in 2014. Given the potential for conflict of interest, it is imperative that today's aspiring physician-scientists be educated regarding the ethics of conducting industry sponsored research and reminded of their Hippocratic oath to serve their patients rather than the interests of a specific third party.[40] Physician-scientists who engage in alternatively sponsored research should have the foresight to predict potential ways in which their results may be exploited or interpreted out of context, and design their studies and manuscripts accordingly to protect the best interests of their patients.

CURRENT OPINIONS AND FUTURE DIRECTIONS

Physician-scientists have the unique potential to combine scientific insight with clinical perspective to advance the field of medicine, either through basic science, outcomes, or health services research. Their cultivation and preservation are critical to maintaining the United States' position as a world leader in biomedical innovation and shaping the future of medicine in an era of rapid change.[23,38] Although previously immune to the pressures that influence other consumer-related service industries, academic medicine in the twenty-first century will be forced to confront declining reimbursements, universal healthcare, direct-to-patient advertising, patient-rated outcomes, exponential growth in technology, structural changes in organization, and regulatory transformations.[23,38] Mastering all of the traditional elements of clinical practice, teaching, research, and administration may not be possible for future physician-scientists, and establishing clinical and research areas of expertise will be critical to achieve academic excellence and leadership in one's surgical field.

For young surgeons today to be successful in developing an academic career, they must understand the aforementioned challenges and prepare themselves for a long and committed road to achieving research independence. They should engage thoughtful mentors who have been successful in their desired research field. Particularly for surgery, these mentors may be in their own surgical field but may also practice in another specialty. Being able to adapt and learn skills from mentors outside of one's specialty may be a critical element for success in certain environments and may also lead to developing innovative collaborative projects worthy of high-profile grants. Residents and junior surgical faculty must also find a way to balance their clinical education with learning the necessary research, administrative, and leadership skills to be competitive. Finally, researchers at all levels must realize at the beginning of their career that triumph over this long path requires an incredible amount of sacrifice and hard work along the way. In the current grim environment for grant success, they should not let negative outcomes lead to a loss of morale or momentum, because with the proper planning and guidance they will persevere.

REFERENCES

1. Dickens C. A tale of two cities. Costa Mesa (CA): Saddleback Publishing; 2011.
2. Rockey S, Collins F. One nation in support of biomedical research. NIH Directors Blog; 2013. Available at: http://directorsblog.nih.gov/2013/09/24/one-nation-in-support-of-biomedical-research/. Accessed December 11, 2013.
3. Davidson NO. Grant writing and academic survival: what the fellow needs to know. Gastrointest Endosc 2005;61(6):726–7.
4. Berger DH. An introduction to obtaining extramural funding. J Surg Res 2005;128(2):226–31.
5. King A, Sharma-Crawford I, Shaaban AF, et al. The pediatric surgeon's road to research independence: utility of mentor-based National Institutes of Health Grants. J Surg Res 2013;184:66–70.
6. Sanfey H, Hollands C. Career development resource: promotion to associate professor. Am J Surg 2012;204:130–4.
7. Sanfey H. Promotion to professor: a career development resource. Am J Surg 2010;200:554–7.
8. The International Campaign to Revitalise Academic Medicine. The future of academic medicine: five scenarios to 2025. New York: Milbank Memorial Fund; 2005. Available at: http://www.milbank.org/uploads/documents/0507FiveFutures/0507FiveFutures.html. Accessed March 17, 2014.
9. Nonnemaker L. Women physicians in academic medicine: new insights from cohort studies. N Engl J Med 2000;342:399–405.
10. Pardes H. The promise and risk of academic medicine. Mayo Clin Proc 2005;80:1349–52.
11. Chen JT, Girotto JA, Kitzmiller WJ, et al. Academic plastic surgery: faculty recruitment and retention. Plast Reconstr Surg 2014;133:393e–404e.
12. Chung KC, Song JW, Kim HM, et al. Predictors of job satisfaction among academic faculty members: do instructional and clinical staff differ? Med Educ 2010;44:985–95.
13. Rangel SJ, Moss RL. Recent trends in the funding and utilization of NIH career development awards by surgical faculty. Surgery 2004;136:232–9.
14. Lai WW, Vetter VL, Richmond M, et al. Clinical research careers: reports from a NHLBI Pediatric Heart Network Clinical Research Skills Development Conference. Am Heart J 2011;161:13–67.
15. Brock MV, Bouvet M. Writing a successful NIH mentored career development grant (K Award): hints for the junior-faculty surgeon. Ann Surg 2010;251(6):1013–7.
16. The Plastic Surgery Foundation Researcher Education Committee. Grant Writing Module. Available at: http://www.thepsf.org/Documents/PSF%20Grant%20Writing%20Module%208.22.13%20FINAL.pdf. Accessed December 15, 2013.
17. Hamilton JG, Birmingham WC, Tehranifar P, et al. Transitioning to independence and maintaining research careers in a new funding climate: American Society of Preventive Oncology Junior Members Interest Group Report. Cancer Epidemiol Biomarkers Prev 2013;22(11):2138–42.
18. Straus SE, Chatur F, Taylor M. Issues in the mentor-mentee relationship in academic medicine: a qualitative study. Acad Med 2009;84:135–9.
19. Zerzan JT, Hess R, Schur E, et al. Making the most of mentors: a guide for mentees. Acad Med 2009;84:140–4.
20. Thoma A, Haines T, Tuku E, et al. How to become a successful clinical investigator. Clin Plast Surg 2008;35(2):305–11.
21. Sackett DL. On the determinants of academic success as a clinician scientist. Clin Invest Med 2001;24:94–100.
22. Boice R. Advice for new faculty members. Nihil Nimus. Toronto: Allyn and Bacon; 2000.
23. Fisherman JA. Matrix mentorship in academic medicine: sustainability of competitive advantage. In: Savage GT, Fottler MD, editors. Biennial review of health care management: MESO perspectives (Advances in Health Care Management, Volume 8). Bingley (United Kingdom): Emerald Group Publishing Limited; 2009. p. 155–70.
24. Franzblau LE, Kotsis SV, Chung KC. Mentorship: concepts and application to training programs. Plast Reconstr Surg 2013;131:837e–43e.
25. Entezami P, Franzblau LE, Chung KC. Surgical mentorship, a systematic review. Hand (N Y) 2012;7:30–6.
26. Lee TH, Ognibene FP, Schwartz JS. Correlates of external research support among respondents to the 1990 American Federation for Clinical Research Survey. Clin Res 1991;39:135–44.
27. Ratcliffe MB, Howard C, Mann M, et al. National Institutes of Health funding for cardiothoracic surgical research. J Thorac Cardiovasc Surg 2008;136:392–7 [discussion: 398–9].

28. Brown AM, Morrow JD, Limbird LE, et al. Centralized oversight of physician-scientist faculty development at Vanderbilt: early outcomes. Acad Med 2008;83:969–75.

29. Inouye SK, Fiellin DA. An evidence based guide to writing grant proposals for clinical research. Ann Intern Med 2005;142:274–82.

30. Chung KC, Shauver MJ. Fundamental principles of writing a successful grant proposal. J Hand Surg Am 2008;33A:566–72.

31. Hanna WC, Mulder DS, Fried GM, et al. Training future surgeons for management roles. Arch Surg 2012;147(10):940–4.

32. Dimick JB. Developing leaders in surgery. Arch Surg 2012;147(10):944–5.

33. Streu R, Hansen J, Abrahamse P, et al. Professional burnout among US plastic surgeons: results of a national survey. Ann Plast Surg 2014;72:346–50.

34. Balch CM, Shanafelt T. Combating stress and burnout in surgical practice: a review. Adv Surg 2010;44:29–47.

35. Shanafelt TD, Boone S, Tan L, et al. Burnout and satisfaction with work-life balance among US physicians relative to the general US population. Arch Intern Med 2012;172:1377–85.

36. Shanafelt TD, Balch CM, Bechamps GJ, et al. Burnout and career satisfaction among American surgeons. Ann Surg 2009;250:463–71.

37. Golub JS, Johns MM, Weiss PS, et al. Burnout in academic faculty of otolaryngology-head and neck surgery. Laryngoscope 2008;118:1951–6.

38. Chapman AB, Guay-Woodford LM. Nurturing passion in a time of academic climate change: the modern day challenge of junior faculty development. Clin J Am Soc Nephrol 2008;3:1878–83.

39. Fox G, Schwartz A, Hart K. Work-family balance and academic advancement in medical schools. Acad Psychiatry 2006;30:227–34.

40. Lundh A, Sismondo S, Lexchin J, et al. Industry sponsorship and research outcome. Cochrane Database Syst Rev 2012;(12):1–91. Available at: http://onlinelibrary.wiley.com/doi/10.1002/14651858.MR000033.pub2/abstract;jsessionid=313F30281550718B2A8405621EEDDC9D.d04t01. Accessed March 17, 2014.

Future Education and Practice Initiatives in Hand Surgery
Improving Fulfillment of Patient Needs

Erika D. Sears, MD, MS*, Kevin C. Chung, MD, MS

KEYWORDS

- Hand surgery training • Competency-based learning • Milestones • Workforce shortages
- Emergency coverage

KEY POINTS

- In the current health care environment, there are several areas in the delivery of health care that need improvement to adequately fulfill the needs of hand surgery patients.
- Some of the areas that require improvement in delivery of health care to patients having hand surgery include shortages in emergency hand call coverage, the decreasing trends in hand surgeons willing to perform microsurgery and replantation, and deficiencies in musculoskeletal education of non–hand surgery providers.
- Both educational reforms and reforms in the practice environment are needed to improve the ability of hand surgeons to fulfill patient needs in the future.

Health services research is not only critical in determining best practices in treatment decisions for patients having hand surgery, but it is also crucial to evaluate areas needing improvement in the process of health care delivery. Several reforms in health care and in the training of physicians make it a challenging environment in which policy makers and leaders must navigate while seeking to improve patient outcomes, satisfaction, and efficient use of limited resources. Challenges that particularly affect the ability to care for patients having hand surgery, both in an emergency and elective setting, include surgical workforce shortages and maldistribution, emergency department overcrowding, decreasing number of trauma centers, uncompensated care, increasing

malpractice costs, and uncertainty of the impact of the Affordable Care Act. At the same time, leaders in academic centers where hand surgeons, orthopedic surgeons, and plastic surgeons are trained must also contend with work hour limitations, limitations in funding and training positions despite workforce shortages, variability in the quality of resident education, and the recent transition of programs toward competency-based and milestone-based curricula.

Many of these reforms and challenges that policy makers face also directly affect the ability of individual physicians to effectively meet the needs of patients having hand surgery. Much attention has been paid to highlighting the difficulty in maintaining subspecialty surgeon coverage for patients

Disclosure: The authors have no financial interest or conflicts of interest to declare in relation to the content of this article.
Support for this study was provided by a Midcareer Investigator Award in Patient-oriented Research (K24 AR053120) to Dr Kevin C. Chung.
Section of Plastic Surgery, Department of Surgery, The University of Michigan Health System, 2130 Taubman Center, SPC 5340, 1500 East Medical Center Drive, Ann Arbor, MI 48109-5340, USA
* Corresponding author.
E-mail address: endavis@med.umich.edu

evaluated in emergency departments. Confining scope of practice has affected the proportion of hand surgeons willing to perform replantation and complex soft tissue reconstruction. In addition, increased attention has highlighted deficiencies in musculoskeletal education of emergency department providers and general practitioners who are often instrumental gatekeepers in deciding which patients are ultimately seen by a hand surgeon.

Not only is it critical for individual providers to fully understand barriers in optimal delivery of care to patients having hand surgery, it is also imperative for providers to be involved in implementing solutions to these challenges despite limitations present in the current health care environment. This article discusses areas of patient care delivery that are in need of improvement based on previous studies in the literature, and highlights potential future initiatives to improve health care delivery and education in hand surgery.

SHORTCOMINGS IN FULFILLMENT OF PATIENT NEEDS
Workforce Shortages

The United States is facing a workforce shortage in the medical community, including surgical specialists.[1,2] Increased coverage of the uninsured and underinsured through the Affordable Care Act is likely to add to the heightened demand for physicians, including hand surgeons. However, no provision in the health care law was made to deal with impending physician shortages. There has been a recent increase in medical school positions, but funding for graduate medical education positions has remained frozen since 1996, despite population growth and expansion of access to health care.[1] These limitations are likely to affect hand surgeons as well as other surgical subspecialties.

No data exist to predict the magnitude of workforce shortages in hand surgery. However, there are predictions of substantial shortages among orthopedic surgeons and plastic surgeons.[1,3,4] Given that these disciplines supply the hand surgeons of the future, it is natural to extrapolate that hand surgery will be similarly affected, especially given that non–Certificate of Added Qualification (CAQ) hand surgeons (non–fellowship-trained plastic and orthopedic surgeons) also provide a great deal of elective and emergency hand surgical care.[5]

Emergency Hand Call Coverage

Hand trauma is the most frequent type of injury treated in emergency departments,[6] but coverage of emergency hand care remains a national problem. Despite research showing profitability in providing hand trauma care,[7] hand surgery is one of the surgical specialties that is most problematic in providing coverage for emergency care; 80% of a national sample of emergency departments reported inadequate hand surgery on-call coverage (**Fig. 1**), second only to plastic surgery (81% reporting inadequate coverage).[8] Alderman and colleagues[7] showed that provision of emergency hand trauma care is financially advantageous to professionals and marginally advantageous to health care facilities, with a profit margin of 25% and 1% respectively. However, the study highlighted that small changes in collection rates or payer mix could easily have negative implications on net revenue. With recent increased coverage of the uninsured through Medicaid expansion and state and federal marketplaces, the resultant impact on profit margins for both emergency and elective hand surgery coverage is unknown and needs to be studied. However, a

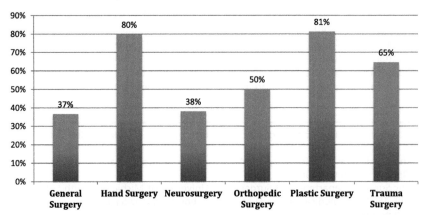

Fig. 1. Percentage of emergency departments from a national sample reporting inadequate on-call coverage by surgical specialty. (*Adapted from* Rao MB, Lerro C, Gross CP. The shortage of on-call surgical specialist coverage: a national survey of emergency department directors. Acad Emerg Med 2010;17:1378; with permission.)

study of the impact of Massachusetts health care reform on payer mix in a tertiary-care orthopedic hand surgery practice found that encounters of uninsured patients decreased from 4% to 2%, whereas encounters of privately insured patients increased from 61% to 65%, and the proportion of encounters with the state Medicaid plan did not change significantly (5.4% before reform vs 5.7% after reform, $P = .143$).[9]

Regardless of potential for profitability, there is reluctance of emergency departments and individual providers to participate in hand call. Some blame the Emergency Medical Treatment and Labor Act (EMTALA) of 1986 not only for the current overcrowding of emergency departments but also for financial challenges prompting many trauma centers across the nation to close, causing an increased reliance on the remaining emergency departments as a safety net for care. The Centers for Medicare and Medicaid Services later clarified EMTALA rules to indicate that hospitals do not have to maintain call coverage for all surgical specialties and left it to their discretion based on their own patient needs and resources.[10] As a result, many hospitals have chosen to decrease call coverage for surgical specialists, either by choice of the facility or by inability to maintain surgeons on staff to cover call as a condition of hospital privileges.

Hand surgeons have increasingly been able to move from the hospital setting to practices purely in the outpatient setting with use of office operating rooms or ambulatory surgery centers. In the state of Tennessee, Anthony and colleagues[11] showed that 37% of the 111 hospitals in the state had hand specialists, but only 24% of hospitals provided coverage of hand specialist call. In addition, although 88% of level-1 trauma centers (7 of 8) in Tennessee had hand specialists, only 25% provided hand specialist call (2 of 8). Similar findings were shown in an evaluation of 3 cities in the state of Florida collectively having more than 30 self-designated hand surgeons, but limited hand surgery emergency call coverage.[12] A single-center study by Kuo and colleagues[13] found that 81% of patients transferred to their center came from emergency departments with partial or full hand surgery call coverage, but only 10% had been evaluated by a hand surgeon before transfer. In addition, a survey of American Society for Surgery of the Hand (ASSH) members found that 29% of respondents reported that they did not take emergency hand call.[14] These studies highlight the discrepancy between hand surgeons having an elective practice and hand surgeons who are willing to cover emergency call.

Several investigators have speculated about the rationale of surgeons limiting their involvement in

hand surgery emergency call, but few data exist to support the conclusions fully. Patients seen in emergency departments are disproportionately uninsured or underinsured.[15] Reimbursement for work performed in the emergency department has been shown to be extremely poor across a range of hospital settings. Collection rates can be as low as 14% and as high as 50% across a range of hospital types.[16] Declining reimbursement in elective practices has made it impractical for hand surgeons to provide a significant amount of uncompensated care in the emergency setting, especially considering costs of malpractice insurance and perceived high risk of litigation in the emergent population, in which there is no established physician-patient relationship. In addition, patients presenting for emergency hand care often present at inconvenient times on evenings or weekends, and patients who present during the day are likely to be disruptive to an elective practice.

Transfer Patterns for Emergency Hand Care

As a result of declining emergency hand call coverage, there has been a great deal of research dealing with the appropriateness of transfers for emergency evaluation by hand surgeons. There is an increased reliance on academic medical centers to serve as a safety net to provide emergency care for patients with hand trauma in addition to other surgical subspecialties. Hand surgeons at receiving facilities often think that many patient transfers are unnecessary.[17] An analysis by Hartzell and colleagues[18] of transfers for emergency hand care found that, although transferred patients were more complex overall, 90% of patients did not have an emergent operation and 27% of patients were discharged directly without a hand surgery consultation. Similar studies found that many transferred patients do not undergo urgent bedside or operative procedures and many do not receive an evaluation by a hand surgery attending.[19,20] In addition, Ozer and colleagues[21] found that 63% of patients transferred via air for evaluation for replantation did not undergo replantation, although one-quarter of these patients chose not to undergo replantation despite being suitable candidates. Air transfers are costly and are a potential source of inefficient use of resources in the care of patients with hand trauma. Dealing with a large number of patients who do not require treatment at a tertiary care facility in addition to caring for patients with complex conditions may put unnecessary strain on these safety-net academic centers.

Given the high number of transfers that are deemed unnecessary, several recent studies have focused on determining whether there are nonmedical characteristics associated with the hand surgery transfer patient population. Data are mixed regarding whether transfer patients are more highly associated with poor insurance status. Several studies have reported that transfer patients were more likely to have no insurance or undesirable insurance (Medicaid or state-sponsored insurance).[17,18,22] However, several other studies found no difference among transferred and nontransferred patients based on insurance status.[13,19,20,23,24] These studies finding no association of poor insurance status in transfer patients concluded that insurance status was likely not the primary driving force behind most transfers. Patients were most likely transferred because of increased complexity of their presenting problem or because of the inability of the referring facility to have patients evaluated by a local hand surgeon.

In addition to putting strain on academic institutions, lack of ability to obtain hand emergency care locally can put undue stresses on patients. Transfers are associated with costs that at times are higher than treatment costs. With some transfer costs not covered by insurance, patients are left with medical bills for which they cannot pay.[17] In addition, lack of local hand surgeons to provide emergency care means that patients have to travel great distances for follow-up care, and, if they are unable to do so for financial reasons, they may be more likely to have subpar outcomes. Calfee and colleagues[25] examined distances that patients traveled to an outpatient tertiary care hand surgery clinic and found that, as distances of required travel increased, the proportion of patients with Medicaid increased steadily. Their Medicaid patients had higher cancellation rates as the distance

traveled increased relative to patients with private insurance traveling similar distances. Thus, transfers not only delay care of patients presenting with hand trauma on the day of injury, but postoperative follow-up is also likely to be a burden on patients transferred lengthy distances.

Replantation and Microsurgical Procedures

A trend toward declining interest in performing replantation and complex microsurgical procedures has been noted in hand surgery,[5,14,26,27] possibly caused by poor reimbursement for time invested or insufficient exposure during training. In an analysis of national data for replantation trends, only 15% of hospitals included in the database in 1996 performed replantation, with only 2% of hospitals performing 10 or more cases during the year.[28] In addition, in 2 separate analyses of national replantation data, an increasing reliance on teaching hospitals to perform replantation was noted, with a declining proportion of replantation being performed in nonteaching hospitals, which was not the case a decade earlier (Fig. 2).[26,29] Peterson and colleagues[30] reported in 2012 that only 55% of all level I trauma centers definitively had a hand surgeon on call willing to accept patients with indications for hand or finger replantation, with only 40% of level I trauma centers having full-time coverage for hand surgery and replantation. A 2007 survey of ASSH members found that 56% of members performed replantations or revascularizations, of whom 13% performed more than 10 per year. Busy elective schedules (51%) and lack of confidence in microsurgical skills (39%) were the most common reasons cited for not performing replantation among

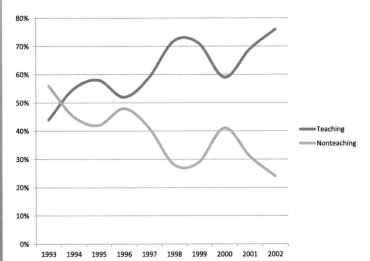

Fig. 2. Percentage of replantations performed based on hospital teaching status. Hospitals with undesignated teaching status are included as nonteaching hospitals. (*Adapted from* Chen MW, Narayan D. Economics of upper extremity replantation: national and local trends. Plast Reconstr Surg 2009;124:2006; with permission.)

these ASSH members. Similar reasons were given among members who did not perform microsurgical procedures.[14]

A discrepancy between the willingness to perform microsurgical procedures in practice has also been noted between surgeons trained in plastic surgery and orthopedic surgery. In a recent role delineation study by Aliu and Chung,[31] respondents from orthopedic hand surgery programs were less likely to think that they had enough exposure for proficiency during training to perform soft tissue reconstruction and microsurgical procedures compared with respondents from plastic surgery programs. These graduates from orthopedic accredited fellowship programs were also less likely to perform microsurgical and soft tissue reconstructive procedures in practice. This role delineation study concluded that differences in exposure of procedures during fellowship training translated to similar limitations in scope of practice after completion of training. Several other studies have noted a tendency of hand surgeons with plastic surgery training backgrounds to think that they are more competent in performing or to be more likely to perform replantation and microsurgical procedures.[14,32,33] Elliott and colleagues[33] found that orthopedic and combined fellowships both offered reasonable exposure to upper extremity microsurgery, but theorized that differences in early microsurgical exposure with plastic surgery residency compared with orthopedic surgery residency made plastic surgeons more likely to perform upper extremity microsurgery on completion of fellowship. In a survey of program directors from orthopedic surgery–accredited and plastic surgery–accredited hand surgery

fellowships, microsurgical procedures were collectively more likely to be rated by plastic surgery programs as essential competencies for graduates to master. However, when only microsurgical nerve procedures were examined, there was no difference in the essential ratings between plastic surgery and orthopedic surgery programs.[34] Thus, the essential nature of microsurgical procedures may be stressed differently among training programs based on orthopedic and plastic surgeon presence.

Plastic surgeons have a decreased presence in hand surgery,[35] being fewer in number and having a lower proportion of graduates obtaining CAQ certification through the American Board of Plastic Surgeons each year (**Figs. 3** and **4**).[36] This trend may ultimately translate to fewer hand surgeons overall being willing to perform reconstructive procedures requiring microsurgical skill.

Musculoskeletal Education of Nonhand Surgeons

Musculoskeletal complaints are the most common reason for patients to see primary care providers,[37] and the upper extremity is the most common site of injury in the emergency department setting.[6] Given the commonality of musculoskeletal complaints, internists, family practitioners, pediatricians, and emergency department physicians should be well versed in the evaluation and management of common upper extremity conditions. However, studies have highlighted limitations in musculoskeletal education in both medical school and residency programs and the resulting deficiencies of general practitioners to effectively

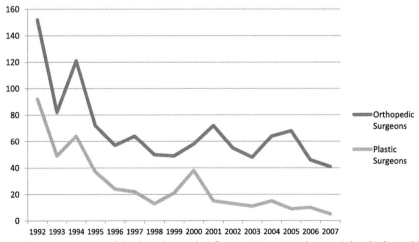

Fig. 3. Number of CAQ in surgery of the hand awarded from 1992 to 2007 by specialty. (*Adapted from* Higgins JP. The diminishing presence of plastic surgeons in hand surgery: a critical analysis. Plast Reconstr Surg 2010;125:252; with permission.)

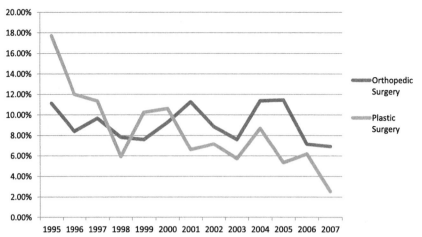

Fig. 4. Percentage of new diplomates in orthopedic surgery and plastic surgery obtaining CAQ in surgery of the hand from 1995 to 2007. (*Adapted from* Higgins JP. The diminishing presence of plastic surgeons in hand surgery: a critical analysis. Plast Reconstr Surg 2010;125:253; with permission.)

manage common hand problems. Freedman and Bernstein[38] found that 78% of recent medical school graduates failed to show basic competency in musculoskeletal medicine according to criteria set independently by internal medicine and orthopedic surgery program directors. An examination of patients referred to a hand surgeon by a primary care provider found that the correct diagnosis was established only 34% of the time. However, the larger problem lies in the realization that 74% of these patients underwent a test or intervention before presenting to a hand surgeon and 70% of these tests or interventions, including expensive imaging modalities, were thought to be unnecessary. In addition, 17% of patients experienced a complication as a result of unnecessary studies or interventions.[39]

Evaluation of medical school curricula across the nation shows little exposure to musculoskeletal medicine, despite the frequency with which musculoskeletal complaints are encountered.[37] Non–hand surgery providers having some degree of exposure to a rotation focusing on musculoskeletal education or orthopedics performed better than students or residents not completing a dedicated rotation.[37,40,41] Deficiencies in the evaluation and management of patients with hand trauma among emergency department providers who first see patients may explain some of the unnecessary transfers of patients for emergency hand care discussed earlier.

EDUCATION INITIATIVES

Several educational initiatives must be advocated for and implemented in order to help overcome many of the challenges discussed in delivery of

care for the hand surgery patient population. It is imperative for hand surgeons to be involved in all realms of medical education, including the training of medical students, plastic surgery residents, orthopedic surgery residents, and hand surgery fellows in order to minimize some of these challenges for future physicians. It is also critical for hand surgeons to be involved in collaborations with primary care disciplines to ensure proper training of non–hand surgery disciplines of relevant aspects within hand surgery with which they should be familiar.

Improvement in Musculoskeletal Education

A solid foundation in musculoskeletal medicine should be required in medical school and built on in residency specialties that see a large number of musculoskeletal conditions. Hand surgeons, orthopedic surgeons, and plastic surgeons must be actively involved in medical school and residency curriculum development to provide critical input into the development of educational endeavors in this domain. Electives and ongoing didactics in musculoskeletal medicine are critical to maintain skills throughout residency training for non–hand surgery providers. Many patients with musculoskeletal complaints are rightfully never seen by a hand surgeon. Thus, it is imperative to adequately prepare trainees to evaluate and manage common upper extremity conditions and know when presenting complaints require referral to a subspecialist.

Plastic and Orthopedic Surgery Residency Training Initiatives

Hand surgeons must be actively involved in training plastic surgery and orthopedic surgery residents and encourage continued active participation of both disciplines in hand surgery. Mentor relationships between faculty and residents are critical in encouraging residents to enter hand surgery.[42] Mentorship and early exposure to hand surgery could help to maintain interest among plastic surgery and orthopedic surgery residents, which is particularly important for plastic surgery training programs because of the diminished presence of plastic surgeons in hand surgery and concern with lack of plastic surgery faculty mentors who are practicing hand surgeons.[36] If plastic surgery residents are unable to have exposure to hand surgery in their home departments, rotations should be sought with orthopedic surgery departments or off site at neighboring institutions that may provide an adequate hand surgery training experience. In orthopedic surgery training programs, residents who have an identified interest in hand surgery should be encouraged to pursue elective plastic surgery rotations in order to offer earlier exposure and develop comfort with microsurgical procedures. In addition, introduction of a microsurgical simulation program could help orthopedic surgery residents have greater comfort in microsurgical techniques earlier in training. These experiences may ultimately improve the willingness and comfort level of orthopedic surgery–trained hand surgeons in performing microsurgical procedures.

Hand Surgery Training Initiatives

A structured competency-based curriculum for hand surgery training should be instituted to provide a comprehensive education in bone and soft tissue facets of hand surgery practices. However, the ability to achieve a standard curriculum requires leadership from the orthopedic and plastic surgery residency review committees, boards, and specialty societies to come together as stakeholders in the process. The Accreditation Council for Graduate Medical Education (ACGME) is taking steps in the right direction in better defining competencies through the Next Accreditation System Milestone Project for each specialty, in which specialty-specific milestones are among the tools used to ensure that fellows are able to practice core professional activities on completion of the program.[43] However, milestones do not represent the entirety of dimensions of the 6 domains (**Box 1**) of physician competency,[44] in which the number of milestones for each specialty in the initial pilot group of 7 specialties ranges from 12 milestones for radiology to 41 milestones for orthopedic surgery.[45] The Milestone Project was piloted for the 7 initial specialties beginning July 2013 and will

---

Box 1
ACGME competency domains

Patient care

Medical knowledge

Practice-based learning and improvement

Interpersonal and communication skills

Professionalism

Systems-based practice

Data from ACGME common program requirements for one-year fellowships. Available at: https://http://www.acgme.org/acgmeweb/Portals/0/PFAssets/ProgramRequirements/One_Year_CPRs_Categorization_07012016.pdf. Accessed March 25, 2014.

---

begin in all other specialties, including hand surgery, in July 2014,[46] with at least semiannual evaluations of residents and fellows to ensure progression through specific milestones. In addition to guiding curriculum development for residents and fellows, milestone evaluations allow continuous monitoring of program outcomes and lengthening of site visit cycles.[47,48]

Even though studies show that orthopedic surgery–accredited hand surgery fellowships generally provide some exposure to microsurgery,[31–33,49] a national survey of hand surgery fellowship program directors found a varying degree of priority placed on microsurgical procedures.[50] In addition, plastic surgery and orthopedic surgery programs have differing opinions as to how essential microsurgical procedures should be for graduates to master.[34] In order to minimize biases introduced by individual hand surgery programs based on primary residency training background, it would be prudent for hand surgery fellows to have exposure to hand surgeons trained in both plastic surgery and orthopedic surgery, ideally through an integrated hand surgery service in which hand surgeons trained in plastic surgery and orthopedic surgery work together and learn from one another. Simulation training could also be used in hand surgery fellowship training to increase exposure to microsurgical techniques, especially in programs that have difficulty in providing adequate exposure to microsurgical procedures because of inadequate case volumes.

PRACTICE INITIATIVES

In addition to educational initiatives, changes in the practice landscape are also warranted to improve challenges in the delivery of care to patients having hand surgery. Hand surgeons must be involved at the local hospital level, regionally, as well as nationally to provide input to improve coordination of trauma care and aid in implementation of strategies to overcome gaps in on-call coverage for hand emergencies.

Incentives for Individual Providers

Physicians cannot be expected to provide extensive uncompensated care in any practice environment given the trend toward declining reimbursement. Although facilities receive subsidies for providing care in underserved areas or providing a disproportionate share of care to uninsured patients, physicians do not receive such direct subsidies.[16] With the Affordable Care Act, some of these subsidies to hospitals will be reduced significantly with the assumption that the number of uninsured patients will decline and the proportion of uncompensated care will decline as a result. Work must be done on a national level to ensure reduction of uncompensated care in the emergency setting if future patient needs are to be met adequately. Hand surgeons must be involved in these policy decisions at the national level.

It is uncertain whether expansion of covered individuals through the Affordable Care Act will be enough incentive to motivate individual providers to participate in on-call responsibilities for patients having hand surgery. Lifestyle issues and impact on elective schedules are also likely to play a large role. However, additional financial incentives such as on-call stipends to compensate surgeons for their time and potential disruption in elective practice may alter the risk/benefit ratio to encourage hand surgeons to provide emergency hand coverage. In addition, incentives such as participation in loan forgiveness programs, the National Health Services Corps, and control of medical malpractice insurance should be considered by the federal government for all physicians practicing in underserved areas rather than focusing solely on providing incentives for primary care providers working in underserved areas, especially because there is a workforce shortage across many medical disciplines.

Coordination of Trauma Care

Much work can be done locally, regionally, and nationally in order to improve coordination of care for patients with hand trauma. In local communities where it is common for hospitals to have partial emergency hand surgery coverage, attempts should be made to coordinate call schedules in order to improve local and regional hand call coverage.

On a regional level, implementation of telemedicine systems may help to reduce the burden from unnecessary transfers. At a minimum, phone consultations with routine transmission of digital photography would be a helpful method of communication between referring and receiving facilities. Telemedicine could allow general practitioners to receive direct advice from hand surgeons regarding appropriate management of patients having hand injury, with the goal of reducing inefficient use of resources and high costs of transportation in unnecessarily transferring low-acuity patients to distant tertiary care centers. In addition, regional centers of excellence for complex hand surgical procedures, such as replantation, could be formally identified to help streamline care for patients with complex hand trauma. If replant centers of excellence are identified, patients could ideally be immediately triaged to these locations in order to reduce temporal delays in receiving care, thereby potentially improving patient outcomes with improved efficiency of care. Additional resources to perform these complex procedures, whether from state or federal sources, should be pooled and directed more efficiently to these centers that perform complex procedures in greater numbers rather than spreading resources inefficiently among other hospitals that perform few complex procedures.

On a national level, development and routine use of transfer guidelines, similar to those guidelines used in trauma[51] and burn care,[52] should be developed for management of patients having hand surgery. Implementation and evaluation of example transfer guidelines for patients having hand surgery transferred into 2 level I trauma centers found that 53% of patients did not require emergent transfer to a level I facility, and that these nonemergent transfers spent a considerably greater amount of time receiving treatment (mean 15.2 hours) compared with patients who were not transferred (mean 3.1 hours).[18] However, additional strategies such as telemedicine and improved musculoskeletal education of emergency providers ideally needs to be implemented in the initial stages to make transfer guidelines an effective and safe strategy for patients on a large scale.

SUMMARY

In the current health care environment, there are several areas in the delivery of health care to patients having hand surgery that need improvement to adequately fulfill patient needs, including difficulty in maintaining adequate emergency call coverage for patients having hand injury, decreasing trends in hand surgeons willing to perform microsurgery and replantation, and deficiencies in musculoskeletal education of non–hand surgery providers. Both educational reforms and reforms in the practice environment are needed to improve the ability of hand surgeons to fulfill patient needs in the future.

REFERENCES

1. Williams TE Jr, Satiani B, Thomas A, et al. The impending shortage and the estimated cost of training the future surgical workforce. Ann Surg 2009;250:590–7.
2. Sheldon GF. Access to care and the surgeon shortage: American Surgical Association forum. Ann Surg 2010;252:582–90.
3. Rohrich RJ, McGrath MH, Lawrence WT, et al. Assessing the plastic surgery workforce: a template for the future of plastic surgery. Plast Reconstr Surg 2010;125:736–46.
4. Yang J, Jayanti MK, Taylor A, et al. The impending shortage and cost of training the future plastic surgical workforce. Ann Plast Surg 2014;72:200–3.
5. Mueller MA, Zaydfudim V, Sexton KW, et al. Lack of emergency hand surgery: discrepancy between elective and emergency hand care. Ann Plast Surg 2012;68:513–7.
6. Niska R, Bhuiya F, Xu J. National Hospital Ambulatory Medical Care Survey: 2007 emergency department summary. Natl Health Stat Report 2010;(26):1–31.
7. Alderman AK, Storey AF, Chung KC. Financial impact of emergency hand trauma on the health care system. J Am Coll Surg 2008;206:233–8.
8. Rao MB, Lerro C, Gross CP. The shortage of on-call surgical specialist coverage: a national survey of emergency department directors. Acad Emerg Med 2010;17:1374–82.
9. Earp BE, Louie D, Blazar P. The impact of Massachusetts health care reform on an orthopedic hand service. J Hand Surg Am 2013;38:2212–7.
10. Bitterman RA. Explaining the EMTALA paradox. Ann Emerg Med 2002;40:470–5.
11. Anthony JR, Poole VN, Sexton KW, et al. Tennessee emergency hand care distributions and disparities: emergent hand care disparities. Hand (N Y) 2013;8:172–8.
12. Caffee H, Rudnick C. Access to hand surgery emergency care. Ann Plast Surg 2007;58:207–8.
13. Kuo P, Hartzell TL, Eberlin KR, et al. The characteristics of referring facilities and transferred hand surgery patients: factors associated with emergency patient transfers. J Bone Joint Surg Am 2014;96:e48.
14. Payatakes AH, Zagoreos NP, Fedorcik GG, et al. Current practice of microsurgery by members of the American Society for Surgery of the Hand. J Hand Surg Am 2007;32:541–7.
15. Pitts SR, Niska RW, Xu J, et al. National Hospital Ambulatory Medical Care Survey: 2006 emergency department summary. Natl Health Stat Report 2008;(7):1–38.
16. Davison SP. Emergency room coverage: an evolving crisis. Plast Reconstr Surg 2004;114:453–7.
17. Friebe I, Isaacs J, Mallu S, et al. Evaluation of appropriateness of patient transfers for hand and microsurgery to a level I trauma center. Hand (N Y) 2013;8:417–21.
18. Hartzell TL, Kuo P, Eberlin KR, et al. The overutilization of resources in patients with acute upper extremity trauma and infection. J Hand Surg Am 2013;38:766–73.
19. Bauer AS, Blazar PE, Earp BE, et al. Characteristics of emergency department transfers for hand surgery consultation. Hand (N Y) 2013;8:12–6.
20. Butala P, Fisher MD, Blueschke G, et al. Factors associated with transfer of hand injuries to a level 1 trauma center: a descriptive analysis of 1147 cases. Plast Reconstr Surg 2014;133:842–8.
21. Ozer K, Kramer W, Gillani S, et al. Replantation versus revision of amputated fingers in patients air-transported to a level 1 trauma center. J Hand Surg Am 2010;35:936–40.
22. Eberlin KR, Hartzell TL, Kuo P, et al. Patients transferred for emergency upper extremity evaluation: does insurance status matter? Plast Reconstr Surg 2013;131:593–600.
23. Melkun ET, Ford C, Brundage SI, et al. Demographic and financial analysis of EMTALA hand patient transfers. Hand (N Y) 2010;5:72–6.
24. Patterson JM, Boyer MI, Ricci WM, et al. Hand trauma: a prospective evaluation of patients transferred to a level I trauma center. Am J Orthop 2010;39:196–200.
25. Calfee RP, Shah CM, Canham CD, et al. The influence of insurance status on access to and utilization of a tertiary hand surgery referral center. J Bone Joint Surg Am 2012;94:2177–84.
26. Chen MW, Narayan D. Economics of upper extremity replantation: national and local trends. Plast Reconstr Surg 2009;124:2003–11.
27. Steyers CM, Chai SH, Blair WF, et al. A role delineation study of hand surgery. J Hand Surg Am 1990;15:681–9.
28. Chung KC, Kowalski CP, Walters MR. Finger replantation in the United States: rates and resource use from the 1996 healthcare cost and utilization project. J Hand Surg Am 2000;25:1038–42.
29. Friedrich JB, Poppler LH, Mack CD, et al. Epidemiology of upper extremity replantation surgery in the United States. J Hand Surg Am 2011;36:1835–40.
30. Peterson BC, Mangiapani D, Kellogg R, et al. Hand and microvascular replantation call availability study: a national real-time survey of level-I and level-II trauma centers. J Bone Joint Surg Am 2012;94:e185.

31. Aliu O, Chung KC. A role delineation study of hand surgery in the USA: assessing variations in fellowship training and clinical practice. Hand (N Y) 2014;9:58–66.

32. Kakar S, Bakri K, Shin AY. Survey of hand surgeons regarding their perceived needs for an expanded upper extremity fellowship. J Hand Surg Am 2012;37:2374–80.e1–3.

33. Elliott RM, Baldwin KD, Foroohar A, et al. The impact of residency and fellowship training on the practice of microsurgery by members of the American Society for Surgery of the Hand. Ann Plast Surg 2012;69:451–8.

34. Sears ED, Larson BP, Chung KC. Program director opinions of core competencies in hand surgery training: analysis of differences between plastic and orthopedic surgery accredited programs. Plast Reconstr Surg 2013;131:582–90.

35. Chang J, Hentz VR, Chase RA. Plastic surgeons in American hand surgery: the past, present, and future. Plast Reconstr Surg 2000;106:406–12.

36. Higgins JP. The diminishing presence of plastic surgeons in hand surgery: a critical analysis. Plast Reconstr Surg 2010;125:248–60.

37. Scher DL, Boyer MI, Hammert WC, et al. Evaluation of knowledge of common hand surgery problems in internal medicine and emergency medicine residents. Orthopedics 2011;34:e279–81.

38. Freedman KB, Bernstein J. Educational deficiencies in musculoskeletal medicine. J Bone Joint Surg Am 2002;84A:604–8.

39. Hartzell TL, Shahbazian JH, Pandey A, et al. Does the gatekeeper model work in hand surgery? Plast Reconstr Surg 2013;132:381e–6e.

40. Lifchez SD. Hand education for emergency medicine residents: results of a pilot program. J Hand Surg Am 2012;37:1245–8.e12.

41. Matzkin E, Smith EL, Freccero D, et al. Adequacy of education in musculoskeletal medicine. J Bone Joint Surg Am 2005;87:310–4.

42. Chung KC, Lau FH, Kotsis SV, et al. Factors influencing residents' decisions to pursue a career in hand surgery: a national survey. J Hand Surg Am 2004;29:738–47.

43. ACGME common program requirements for one-year fellowships. Available at: https://http://www.acgme.org/acgmeweb/Portals/0/PFAssets/ProgramRequirements/One_Year_CPRs_Categorization_07012016.pdf. Accessed March 25, 2014.

44. ACGME: The Hand Surgery Milestone Project. Available at: http://acgme.org/acgmeweb/Portals/0/PDFs/Milestones/HandSurgeryMilestones.pdf. Accessed March 25, 2014.

45. Swing SR, Beeson MS, Carraccio C, et al. Educational milestone development in the first 7 specialties to enter the next accreditation system. J Grad Med Educ 2013;5:98–106.

46. ACGME: key dates for phase I and phase II specialties operating under the next accreditation system. Available at: https://http://www.acgme.org/acgmeweb/Portals/0/PDFs/NAS/KeyDatesPhase1specialties.pdf. Accessed March 25, 2014.

47. Nasca TJ, Philibert I, Brigham T, et al. The next GME accreditation system–rationale and benefits. N Engl J Med 2012;366:1051–6.

48. ACGME: milestones. Available at: https://http://www.acgme.org/acgmeweb/tabid/430/ProgramandInstitutionalAccreditation/NextAccreditationSystem/Milestones.aspx. Accessed March 25, 2014.

49. Sears ED, Larson BP, Chung KC. Gaps in exposure to essential competencies in hand surgery fellowship training: a national survey of program directors. Hand (N Y) 2013;8:1–11.

50. Sears ED, Larson BP, Chung KC. A national survey of program director opinions of core competencies and structure of hand surgery fellowship training. J Hand Surg Am 2012;37:1971–7.e7.

51. Guidelines for trauma care systems. American College of Emergency Physicians. Ann Emerg Med 1987;16:459–63.

52. Hospital and prehospital resources for optimal care of patients with burn injury: guidelines for development and operation of burn centers. American Burn Association. J Burn Care Rehabil 1990;11:98–104.

Index

Note: Page numbers of article titles are in **boldface** type.

A

Accountable care organizations, 349, 350

Accreditation Council for Graduate Medical Education, competency domains, 383

Affordable Care Act, access to, 346–348
  cost of, 348
  goals and components of, 346
  impact on hand surgeons, 350
  key aspects of, 346–349
  patient protection and, primer for hand surgeons, **345–352**
  quality of, US Centers for Medicare and Medicare Services and, 348–349
  tax increases caused by, 350
  ten titles of, 346, 347

American Board of Plastic Surgeons, Certificate of Added Qualification and, 381, 382

Antibiotics, during elective hand surgery, 270

Arm, Shoulder and Hand, Disabilities of, patient questionnaire, 331

Arthritis, basilar joint, of thumb, 272–273

B

Bench to bedside, integrating advances in basic science into daily clinical practice, **305–317**

C

Career development pathway, mapping of, 369–371

Career management, 373–374

Carpal tunnel, steroid injections into, 275

Carpal tunnel release, postoperative splinting after, 271–272

Casting, versus external fixation, in distal radius fractures, 276–277

Certificate of Added Qualification, American Board of Plastic Surgeons and, 381, 382

Clinical practice guidelines, **361–365**
  in hand surgery, development of, 361
  why physicians do not use, 362–363

Collaborative quality improvement, 336–337
  conceptual model of, 337
  in surgery, **335–343**
  key elements of, 337, 338

Company(ies), new, starting of, 310–314
    business plan for, 311–313
    funding for, 313–314
    startup, composition of, 312, 313
      problems of, 309, 312
      technology transfer office licensing for, 310

Comparative effectiveness research, challenges in, 324–326
  database, and multi-institutional randomized controlled trials compared, 321
  definition of, 320
  electronic databases in, value of, 320–322
  in hand surgery, 322
  incorporating patient-reported outcome measures into, 322
  methodology of, 320
  musculoskeletal-related, federal grants for, 324, 325
  US Institute of Medicine and, 319–320
  used in observational database methodologies, 323

Consumer Assessment of Healthcare Providers and Systems, 332

Cubital syndrome, surgical treatment of, 272

D

Dupuytren contracture, patient education material for, 357

Dupuytren disease, metacarpophalangeal joint contracture in, 286

E

Endoscopic surgery, versus open surgery, for carpal tunnel release, 274–275

Epicondylitis, lateral, treatment of, evidence-based medicine in, 269–270

Evidence-based medicine, importance in clinical practice, 285
  in hand surgery, 285–286
  in treatment of lateral epicondylitis, 269–270

F

Flexor tendon injuries, zone II, repair of, 270–271

Food and Drug Administration, obtaining clearance from, 314–315
    for medical devices, 314–315
    for tissue-engineering medical products, 315

hand.theclinics.com

G

Good manufacturing practices facility, production in, 315
Grant(s), career development, federally funded mentored, 371
  funding of, and promotional tenure, changing climate of, 374
  types of, 371, 372
  writing and submitting of, 371–373

H

Hand, function of, core sets of content related to, patient-reported outcome measures and, 299–300
Hand care, emergency, transfer patterns for, 379–380
Hand surgeons, Affordable Care Act patient protection and primer for, **345–352**
  impact of Affordable Care Act on, 350
Hand surgery, comparative effectiveness research in, **319–327**
  cost/benefit ratio of, 330–331
  development of clinical practice guidelines in, 361
  education initiatives and, 382–383
  elective, antibiotics in, 270
  evidence-based medicine in, **269–283**, 285–286
    failure to unify consensus on treatment in, 273–276
    to unify treatment strategies, 269–272
    where it is still out, 276–279
  functional recovery after, 330–331
  future education and practice initiatives in, **377–386**
  health-related quality of life following, 331
  health services research in, 264
  patient-centered care in, guidelines for, 355–357
  patient-reported outcome instruments in, 290
  patient-reported outcomes of, **293–304**
  patient-reported outcomes relevant to, examples of, 296
  practice initiatives in, 383–384
  quality assessment in, **329–334**
  replantation and microsurgical procedures in, 380–381
  training initiatives and, 383
  treatment effectiveness in, benefits versus potential costs of, 291
    benefits versus potential harm and, 290–291
    measuring and understanding of, **285–292**
Hand trauma, care in, coordination of, 384
  treated in emergency department, 378–379
Health care costs, in United States, 332
Health care reform, in United States, 345
Health services research, aspects of, 260–262
  definition of, 260
  evolution and applications of, **259–268**

examples of, 261
framework of, 262
history of, 259–260
in hand surgery, 264
in surgery, 263–264
  patient engagement in, 264
  postoperative outcomes of, measurement of, 263–264
  variation in care, 263

L

Leahy-Smith America Invents Act, 308

M

Marketing and licensing, with technology transfer office, 310–314
Medical devices, clinical trials with, 315–316
  Food and Drug Administration clearance for, obtaining of, 315
Medical workforce shortages, 378
Medicine, and surgery, patient-centered care in, **353–359**
Metacarpophalangeal joint arthroplasty, in rheumatoid arthritis, 276
Musculoskeletal education, 382
  of nonhand surgeons, 381–382

O

Open surgery, versus endoscopic surgery, for carpal tunnel release, 274–275

P

Patent filing, technology transfer office and, 310–314
Patent protection, definition and purpose of, 307–308
Patents, application, marketing and licensing of, 309
  specifications of, 309, 311
  for scientific discovery, intricacies of, 307–309
  international, 308
  provisional application, 308
  requirements for, 308–309
  steps in obtaining, 309
  types of, 308
Patient-centered care, and evidence-based medicine, balancing of, 355
  five care components of, 354
  in hand surgery, guidelines for, 355–357
  in medicine and surgery, **353–359**
  progression from paternalism to, 353–354
  versus disease-centered care, 354–355
Patient-Centered Outcome Research Institute, priorities and criteria of, 349
Patient encounters, face-to-face, time spent in, maximizing of, 355–356

involving patients in their care, 356–357

nonmedical aspects of, documenting of, 356

patient education material for, 357

Patient needs, fulfillment of, shortcomings in, 378–382

Patient outcomes, after hand surgery, 330–331

Patient-reported outcome measures, 293–294

computer-adaptive testing and, 300–301

computerized forms of, 300

consensus on core constructs, 300

core sets of content related to hand function, 299–300

implementation of, 294

in clinical practice, advantages and limitations of, 297–298

incorporation into comparative effectiveness research, 322

innovations in measurement of, 299–301

interpretation of, in individual patients, information needed for, 298

scores, application to individual patients, 298–299

Patient-reported outcome(s), administration format, 295

generic versus condition-specific instruments, 295

in clinical research, advantages and limitations in, 295–297

of hand surgery, **293–304**

relevant to hand surgery, examples of, 296

Patient-Reported Outcomes Measurement Information System, 331

Physician/scientist pyramid for success, 369, 370

Physicians, changing practices, how and why, 363–364

Plastic and orthopedic surgery residency training initiatives, 382–383

Plastic surgeons, Certificate of Added Qualification and, 381, 382

Platelet-rich plasma, utility of, in tendinopathy and tendon injury, 275–276

Pronator quadratus repair, after distal radius surgery, 273–274

Q

Quality assessment improvement models, pay for, versus pay for performance, 336

Quality assessment metrics, 329

Quality collaborative(s), challenges of, 341

critical elements of, 337–338

improvement programs, advantages of, 340–341

clinical data provided through, 339

future directions in, 341

in practice: Michigan experience, 338–340

in bariatric surgery, 339–340

in cardiac surgery, 339

in general and vascular surgery, 340

in trauma surgery, 340

Quality of care, in United States, 335

R

Radius, distal, fractures of, cast versus external fixation in, 276–277

surgery of, pronator quadratus repair after, 273–274

Randomized clinical trial, clinically important outcomes of, 289–290

inclusion and exclusion criteria of, 289

results of, application to patient care, 289–291

treatment effectiveness in, results of, clinical significance of, 288–289

understanding of, 286, 288

Randomized controlled trial, key features of, 287

methodology of, assessment of, 286

multi-institutional, and comparative effectiveness research database, compared, 321

Research, choosing of research mentor for, 368–369

funding of, current options and future directions in, 374–375

in twenty-first century, **367–376**

Rheumatoid arthritis, metacarpophalangeal joint arthroplasty in, 276

S

Scaphoid fractures, nondisplaced, management of, 277–278

Scientific discovery, partnering with technology transfer office and, 306

patenting of, intricacies of, 307–309

Splinting, postoperative, after carpal tunnel release, 271–272

Steroid injections, into carpal tunnel, 275

Surgeons, career path for, 370

nonhand, musculoskeletal education of, 381–382

Surgery, and medicine, patient-centered care in, **353–359**

collaborative quality improvement in, **335–343**

Surgery quality measures, ambulatory, of US Centers for Medicare and Medicaid Services, 330

Surgical care, quality of, strategies to improve, 335–336

variation in, in United States, 335

Surgical safety, 329–333

T

Technology transfer office, and patent filing, 308

licensing for startup companies, 310

marketing and licensing with, 309–310

partnering with, after scientific discovery, 306

role of, and technology transfer process, 306–307

starting company and, 310–314

Tendinopathy and tendon injury, platelet-rich plasma
    in, 275–276
Thumb, basilar joint arthritis of, 272–273
Tissue-engineering medical products, clinical trials
    with, 316
    Food and Drug Administration clearance for,
        obtaining of, 315
Treatment effectiveness. See also *Hand surgery,
    treatment effectiveness in.*
    in randomized controlled trial, results of, clinical
        significance of, 288–289

understanding of, 286–289
    interpretation of, important concepts in, 286–289
Treatment strategies, evidence-based medicine in
    hand surgery, to unify, 276–279
Trials, randomized. See *Randomized clinical trial,
    Randomized controlled trial.*

U

US Institute of Medicine, and comparative
    effectiveness research, 319–320

Printed and bound by CPI Group (UK) Ltd, Croydon, CR0 4YY

03/10/2024

01040381-0010